# Keto Diet Cookbook In 5

## BY

## Henry Liaw



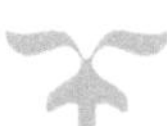

# Subtitle: -

# A Practical Approach to Health: Lose Weight & Lower Blood Sugar Levels, Prevent & Reverse Type 2 Diabetes Naturally

# DISCLAIMER

The recipes and information in this book are provided for educational purposes only. Please always consult a licensed professional before making changes to your lifestyle or diet. The author and publisher shall have neither liability nor responsibility to anyone with respect to any loss or damage caused or alleged to be caused directly or indirectly by the information contained in this book.

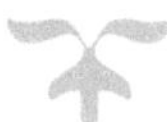

# TABLE OF CONTENT

*HERBED CREAM CHEESE OMELET*

*BABY SPINACH OMELET*

*SAUSAGE, EGG, AND CHEESE SCRAMBLE*

*EASY CLOUD BREAD*

*VEGGIE POACHED EGGS*

*HAM AND CHEESE CHOP*

*EGG WHITE OMELET*

*CORNED BEEF HASH CAKES*

*GREEN CHILI CASSEROLE*

*LOW-CARB KETO BREAKFAST MUFFINS*

*VEGAN QUINOA OATMEAL*

*SPICY PORK SAUSAGE*

*SAUSAGE CHEESE BALLS*

## LUNCH

*CRAB SALAD*

*HAM SPREAD*

*HAM AND CHEESE SALAD*

*EGG SALAD*

*FRESH LOBSTER SALAD*

*VEGETARIAN SANDWICH SPREAD*

*HEALTHIER BBQ PORK FOR SANDWICHES*

*VIRGINA'S TUNA SALAD*

*CHICKEN SALAD SPREAD*

*SUSHI-INSPIRED TUNA SALAD*

*SAVORY STUFFED CELERY BITES*

*BLACKBERRY SPINACH SALAD*

*FETA-STUFFED HAMBURGERS*

*CHICKEN WALNUT CHEESE WRAPPED IN BACON*

*PEACHY CHICKEN SALAD*

*CHIPOTLE BLUE CHEESE DIP*

*SPINACH SALAD WITH EASE*

*CURRY CHICKEN SALAD*

*LOOSEMEAT SANDWICHES II*

*BOLOGNA SALAD SANDWICH SPREAD*

*PESTO TUNA SALAD WITH SUN-DRIED TOMATOES*

*CRAB LEGS WITH GARLIC BUTTER SAUCE*

*BEER BRATS*

*SLOW COOKER MACHACA*

*PINWHEELS*

*PICKLE ROLLUPS*

*HUMMUS*

*VEGETABLE BEEF SOUP WITH GROUND BEEF*

*BROILED SALMON PESTO*

# DINNER

*SLOW COOKER POT ROAST*

*GARLIC CHICKEN*

*SLOW COOKER PULLED PORK*

*MAPLE SALMON*

*SALSA CHICKEN*

*ZESTY SLOW COOKER CHICKEN BARBECUE*

*LOW-CAL CHICKEN*

*BBQ PORK FOR SANDWICHES*

*GARLIC CHICKEN LIVERS*

*GARLIC PRIME RIB*

*BBQ RIBS*

*JUICY ROASTED CHICKEN*

*FOOLPROOF RIB ROAST*

*PUFFS*

*CREAM DILL SAUCE*

*SHRIMP SCAMPI BAKE*

*MOCK SLIDERS*

*SARGE'S EZ PULLED PORK BBQ*

*FESTIVE ONIONS*

*CHICKEN GIZZARDS*

*MUSTARD CREAM SAUCE*

*SEARED CATFISH CREOLE*

*KALUA PORK*

*SOFT SPREAD BUTTER*

*CHICKEN ON A STICK*

*GREEN TURKEY AND CHEESE CASSEROLE*

*MARINATED CHICKEN BARBECUE*

*SAVORY SPINACH CASSEROLE*

*HEALTHIER HOT LEGS*

*GREEN CHICKEN*

## DESSERT

*KETO AVOCADO DESSERT*

*KETO CHOCOLATE MOUSSE*

*90-SECOND KETO BREAD IN A MUG*

*CAULIFLOWER KETO CASSEROLE*

*NO-CHURN KETO ICE CREAM*

*TASTY COLLARD GREENS*

*SAUSAGE STUFFED JALAPENOS*

*GRILLED ASPARAGUS*

*PRETZEL TURTLES*

*PUMPKIN PIE SPICE I*

*HOMESTYLE TURKEY, THE MICHIGANDER WAY*

*FABULOUS BEEF TENDERLOIN*

*ROASTED GARLIC CAULIFLOWER*

*PINA COLADA COOKIES I*

*PUMPKIN SPICE*

*RAW CANDY*

*PUMPKIN COOKIE DIP*

*POPCORN MACAROONS*

*MINI MERINGUES*

*GET WELL CUSTARD*

*KETO PEANUT BUTTER COOKIES*

*KETO PEANUT COOKIES*

*CREAM PUFF SHELLS*

*CREAM CHEESE TART SHELLS*

*LOW CARB FLAVORED MERINGUE COOKIES*

*PUDDING COOKIES I*

*CHEWY KETO CHOCOLATE COOKIES*

*FAUX CHOCOLATE MOUSSE*

*PEANUT BUTTER CHOCOLATE COOKIES*

*KETO PEANUT BUTTER FUDGE FAT BOMB*

## DRINKS

*GREEN LEMONADE*

*HONEY LEMON TEA*

*FRIENDSHIP TEA*

*SMOOTH SWEET TEA*

*ICED LEMON COFFEE*

*PALEO AND KETO ALMOND BUTTER MOCHA FOR TWO*

*BREAKFAST ZINGER JUICE*

*CARROT AND ORANGE JUICE*

*BREAKFAST IN BANGKOK*

*BEER MARGARITAS*

*FUSS FREE HOT CRANBERRY TEA*

*WATERMELON AGUA FRESCA*

*CELYNE'S GREEN JUICE*

*SIMPLE SYRUP*

*BEVERAGE CUBES*

*BOSTON ICED TEA*

*ORANGE SPICE TEA MIX*

*WATERMELON AND BELL PEPPER SLUSH*

*INSTANT RUSSIAN TEA*

*CUCUMBER COOLER*

*SPICED TEA MIX*

*CUCUMBER TEA SPRITZER*

*THAI ICED TEA (CHA YEN)*

*COCOA TEA MIX RECIPE*

*WATERMELON SUMMERTIME SLUSH*

*CHOCOLATE-Y ICED MOCHA*

*SPRINGTIME CITRUS COOLER*

*SOUTH CAROLINA SWEET TEA*

*RUSSIAN TEA II*

*KUWAITI TRADITIONAL TEA*

# COPYRIGHT

In no way is it legal to reproduce, duplicate, or transmit any part of this document in either electronic means or in printed format. Recording of this publication is strictly prohibited and any storage of this document is not allowed unless with written permission from the publisher. All rights reserved.

The information provided herein is stated to be truthful and consistent, in that any liability, in terms of inattention or otherwise, by any usage or abuse of any policies, processes, or directions contained within is the solitary and utter responsibility of the recipient reader. Under no circumstances will any legal responsibility or blame be held against the publisher for any reparation, damages, or monetary loss due to the information herein, either directly or indirectly.

Respective authors own all copyrights not held by the publisher. The information herein is offered for informational purposes solely, and is universal as so. The presentation of the information is without contract or any type of guarantee assurance.

The trademarks that are used are without any consent, and the publication of the trademark is without permission or backing by the trademark owner. All trademarks and brands within this book are for clarifying purposes only and are the owned by the owners themselves, not affiliated with this document.

# INTRODUCTION TO KETO DIET

Are you interested in losing weight? Are you tired of diets that advocate low or no fats and crave your high fat meats? You may well be considering going on the keto diet, the new kid on the block. Endorsed by many celebrities including Halle Berry, LeBron James and Kim Kardashian among others, the keto diet has been the subject of much debate among dietitians and doctors. Do you wonder if the keto diet is safe and right for you?

## WHAT IS THE KETOGENIC DIET ANYWAY?

You must be aware that the body uses sugar in the form of glycogen to function. The keto diet that is extremely restricted in sugar forces your body to use fat as fuel instead of sugar, since it does not get enough sugar. When the body does not get enough sugar for fuel, the liver is forced to turn the available fat into ketones that are used by the body as fuel - hence the term ketogenic.

This diet is a high fat diet with moderate amounts of protein. Depending on your carb intake the body reaches a state of ketosis in less than a week and stays there. As fat is used instead of sugar for fuel in the body, the weight loss is dramatic without any supposed restriction of calories.

The keto diet is such that it you should aim to get 60-75% of your daily calories from fat, 15-30% from protein and only 5-10% from

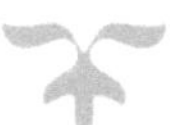

carbohydrates. This usually means that you can eat only 20-50 grams of carbs in a day.

## WHAT CAN YOU EAT ON THIS DIET?

The diet is a high fat diet that is somewhat similar to Atkins. However, there is greater emphasis on fats, usually 'good' fats. On the keto diet you can have

- Olive oil
- Coconut oil
- Nut oils
- Butter
- Ghee
- Grass fed beef
- Chicken
- Fish
- Other meats
- Full fat cheese
- Eggs
- Cream
- Leafy greens
- Non-starchy vegetables
- Nuts
- Seeds

You can also get a whole range of snacks that are meant for keto followers. As you can see from this list, fruits are restricted. You can have low sugar fruits in a limited quantity (mostly berries), but will have to forego your favorite fruits as these are all sweet and/or starchy.

This diet includes no grains of any kind, starchy vegetables like potatoes (and all tubers), no sugar or sweets, no breads and cakes, no beans and lentils, no pasta, no pizza and burgers and very little alcohol. This also means no coffee with milk or tea with milk - in fact, no milk and ice-creams and milk based desserts.

Many of these have workarounds as you can get carbohydrate free pasta and pizza, you can have cauliflower rice and now there are even restaurants that cater to keto aficionados.

## WHAT ARE THE BENEFITS OF THE KETO DIET?

If you are wondering if this diet is safe, its proponents and those who have achieved their weight loss goals will certainly agree that it is safe. Among the benefits of the keto diet you can expect:

- Loss of weight
- Reduced or no sugar spikes
- Appetite control
- Seizure controlling effect
- Blood pressure normalizes in high blood pressure patients

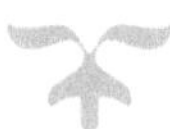

- Reduced attacks of migraine
- Type 2 diabetes patients on this diet may be able to reduce their medications
- Some benefits to those suffering from cancer

Apart from the first four, there is not sufficient evidence to support its effectiveness or otherwise for other diseases as a lot more research is required over the long-term.

## ARE THERE ANY SIDE-EFFECTS OF THIS DIET?

When you initially start the keto diet, you can suffer from what is known as keto flu. These symptoms may not occur in all people and usually start a few days after being on the diet, when your body is in a state of ketosis. Some of the side-effects are:

- Nausea
- Cramps and tummy pain
- Headache
- Vomiting
- Diarrhea and/or constipation
- Muscle cramps
- Dizziness and poor concentrations
- Insomnia
- Carbohydrate and sugar cravings

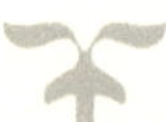

These may take up to a week to subside as your body get used to the new diet regime. You can also suffer from other problems when you start the keto diet - you may find that you have increased urination, so it is important to keep yourself well hydrated. You may also suffer from keto breath when your body reaches optimal ketosis and you can use a mouthwash or brush your teeth more frequently.

Usually the side effects are temporary and once your body acclimatizes to the new diet, these should disappear.

## HOW SAFE IS THE KETO DIET?

Just like any other diet that restricts foods in specific categories, the keto diet is not without risks. As you are not supposed to eat many fruits and vegetables, beans and lentils and other foods, you can suffer from lack of many essential nutrients. Since the diet is high in saturated fats and, if you indulge in the 'bad' fats, you can have high cholesterol levels upping your risk of heart disease.

In the long-term the keto diet can also cause many nutritional deficiencies since you cannot eat grains, many fruits and vegetables and miss out on fiber as also important vitamins, minerals, phytonutrients and antioxidants among other things. You can suffer from gastrointestinal distress, lowered bone density (no dairy and other sources of calcium) and kidney and liver problems (the diet puts added stress on both the organs).

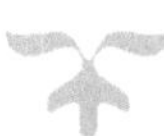

# IS THE KETO DIET SAFE FOR YOU?

If you are willing to forego your usual dietary staples and are really keen to lose weight, you may be tempted to try out the keto diet. The biggest issue with this diet is poor patient compliance thanks to the carbohydrate restriction, so you have to be sure that you can live with your food choices. If you simply find it too difficult to follow, you can go on a version of the modified keto diet that offers more carbs.

However, the keto diet is definitely effective in helping you lose weight. According to a recent study many of the obese patients followed were successful in losing weight. Any problems that they faced were temporary. If you do not have any significant health problems except for obesity and have been unsuccessful in losing weight following any conventional diet, the keto diet may a viable option. You must be absolutely determined to lose the weight and be prepared to go on a restricted diet as specified. Even if you have any medical problems, you can take your doctor's advice and a nutritionist's guidance and go on this diet.

Another study that was carried out for a longer time showed that going on the keto diet is beneficial in weight loss and also results in reduced cholesterol levels with a decrease in the bad cholesterol and an increase in the good cholesterol.

Is the keto diet safe for you? Most doctors and nutritionists are agreed that the keto diet is good for weight loss over the short-term. As for the long-term, more studies are needed. Do keep in mind that obesity is not an apt choice as it comes with its own risk of health problems.

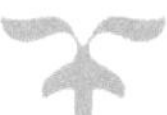

# BREAKFAST

# BASIC CREPES

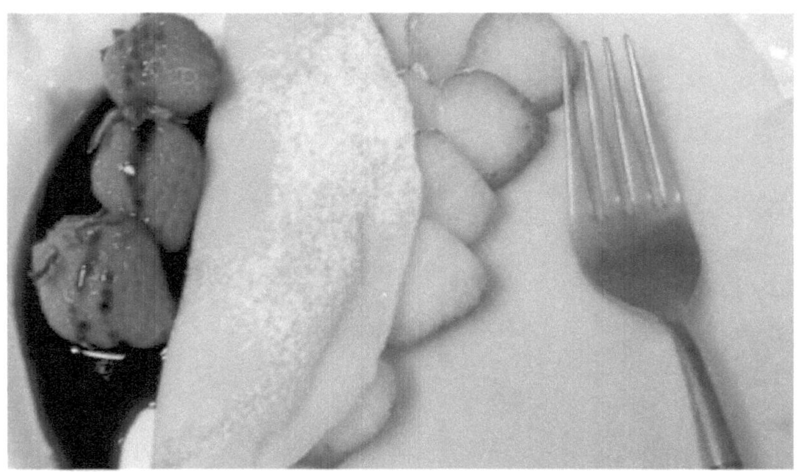

"Here is a simple but delicious crepe batter which can be made in minutes. It's made from ingredients that everyone has on hand."

## INGREDIENTS

- 1 cup all-purpose flour
- 2 eggs
- 1/2 cup milk and water
- 1/4 teaspoon salt
- 2 tablespoons butter, melted

# DIRECTIONS

Prep
10 m

Cook
20 m

Ready In
30 m

Servings
4

- In a large mixing bowl, whisk together the flour and the eggs. Gradually add in the milk and water, stirring to combine. Add the salt and butter; beat until smooth.
- Heat a lightly oiled griddle or frying pan over medium high heat. Pour or scoop the batter onto the griddle, using approximately 1/4 cup for each crepe. Tilt the pan with a circular motion so that the batter coats the surface evenly.
- Cook the crepe for about 2 minutes, until the bottom is light brown. Loosen with a spatula, turn and cook the other side. Serve hot.

# NUTRITION FACTS

Per Serving: 216 calories; 9.2 g fat; 25.5 g carbohydrates; 7.4 g protein; 111 mg cholesterol; 235 mg sodium.

# FRENCH TOAST

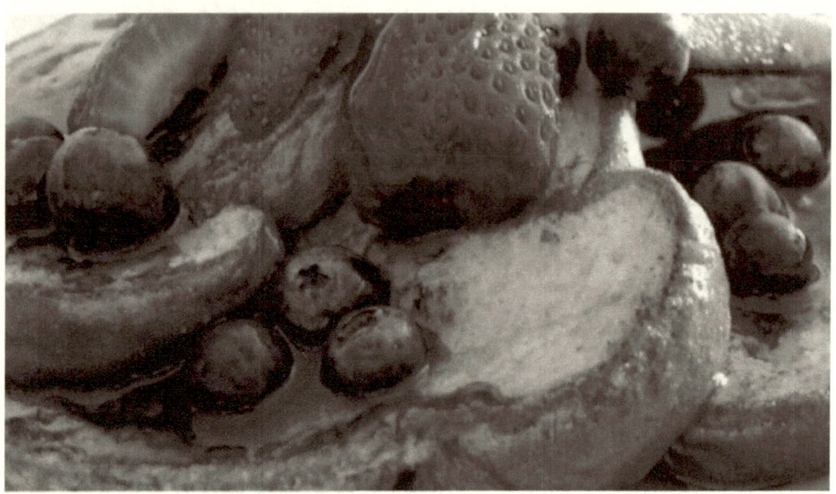

"There are many, fancy variations on this basic recipe. This recipe works with many types of bread - white, whole wheat, cinnamon-raisin, Italian or French. Serve hot with butter or margarine and maple syrup."

## INGREDIENTS

- 6 thick slices bread
- 2 eggs
- 2/3 cup milk
- 1/4 teaspoon ground cinnamon (optional)
- 1/4 teaspoon ground nutmeg (optional)
- salt to taste

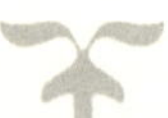

# DIRECTIONS

Prep
5 m

Cook
15 m

Ready In
20 m

Servings
3

- Beat together egg, milk, salt, desired spices and vanilla.
- Heat a lightly oiled griddle or skillet over medium-high heat.
- Dunk each slice of bread in egg mixture, soaking both sides. Place in pan, and cook on both sides until golden. Serve hot.

# NUTRITION FACTS

Per Serving: 240 calories; 6.4 g fat; 33.6 g carbohydrates; 10.6 g protein; 128 mg cholesterol; 478 mg sodium.

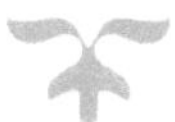

# SPINACH QUICHE WITH COTTAGE CHEESE

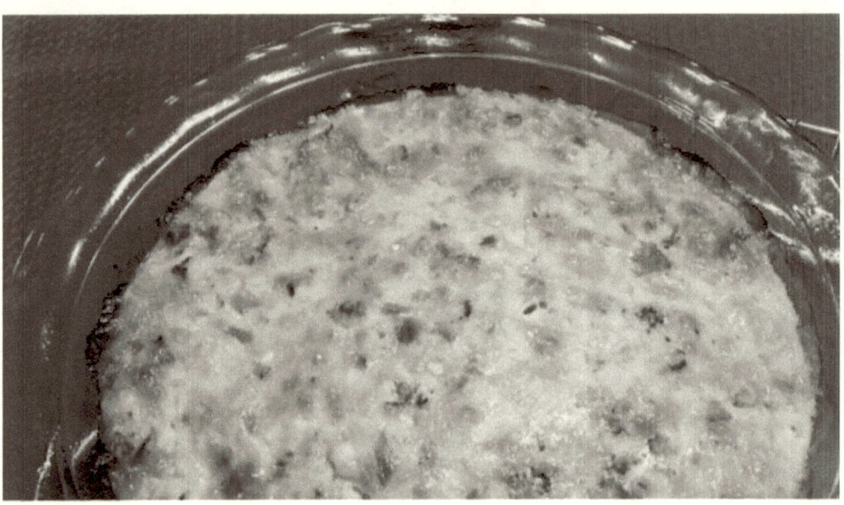

Without a doubt, the number one recipe on Stylish Spoon is my recipe for crustless spinach quiche. It has the most hits, has been featured on other sites the most of any post on this site, and so many of close friends make this crustless quiche for themselves.

## INGREDIENTS

- 1 (10 ounce) package frozen chopped spinach, thawed
- 1 bunch green onions, finely chopped (white parts only)
- 1 (16 ounce) package cottage cheese
- 2 cups shredded Cheddar cheese,    4 eggs, beaten
- 1/4 cup crushed croutons

# DIRECTIONS

Prep
10 m

Cook
1 h

Ready In
1 h 10 m

Servings
8

- Preheat oven to 325 degrees F (165 degrees C). Lightly grease a 9 inch pie or quiche pan.
- Place spinach in a small saucepan. Cook over medium heat, stirring occasionally until soft. Drain off any remaining liquid. Stir in green onions, eggs, cottage cheese and Cheddar cheese. Pour mixture into prepared pan.
- Bake uncovered in preheated oven for 45 minutes. Remove from oven and sprinkle with crushed croutons. Return to oven and bake for an additional 15 minutes, until eggs are set.

# NUTRITION FACTS

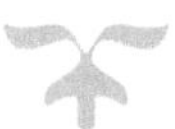

Per Serving: 231 calories; 14.9 g fat; 6.1 g carbohydrates; 19.1 g protein; 131 mg cholesterol; 478 mg sodium.

# BAKING POWDER BISCUITS

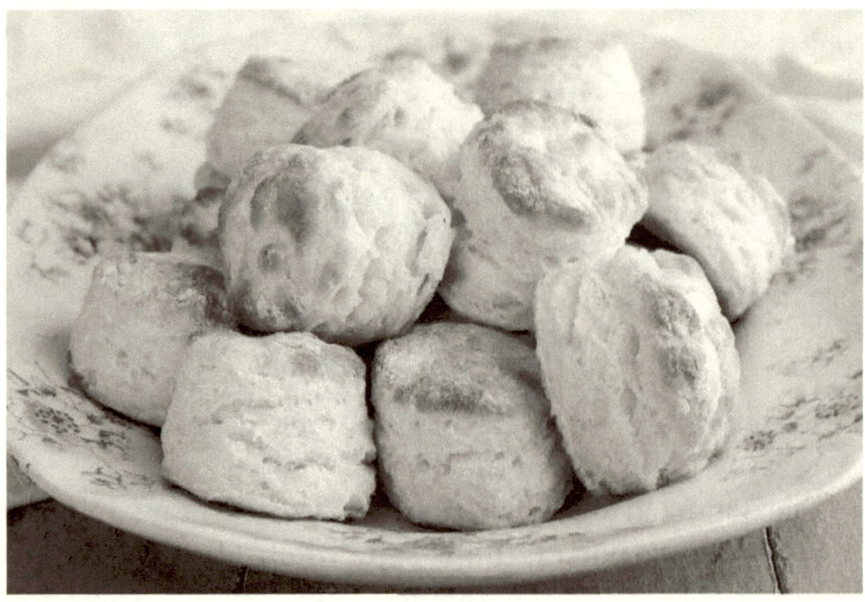

Biscuits are a classic American treat. Mix together just a few simple ingredients and in less than 30 minutes, you can have fresh, warm biscuits on the table — perfect for a leisurely breakfast, savory supper, or served with jam and a cup of afternoon tea.

# INGREDIENTS

- 1/3 cup all-purpose flour
- 1/2 teaspoon baking powder
- 1/8 teaspoon salt
- 2-1/2 teaspoons shortening
- 2 tablespoons milk

# DIRECTIONS

Prep
15 m

Cook
15 m

Ready In
30 m

Servings
4

- Preheat your oven to 425°F with a rack in the upper portion. Get out a baking sheet; there's no need to grease it. Line it with parchment if you like, for easiest cleanup.

- Weigh your flour; or measure it by gently spooning it into a cup, then sweeping off any excess.

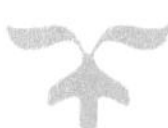

- Mix together the flour, salt, baking powder, and sugar.

- Work the butter into the flour mixture using your fingers, a fork or pastry blender, a stand mixer, or a food processor; your goal is an evenly crumbly mixture (think breadcrumbs).

- Drizzle the smaller amount of milk evenly over the flour mixture. Mix quickly and gently for about 15 seconds, until you've made a cohesive dough. If the mixture seems dry and won't come together, don't keep working it; drizzle in enough milk — up to an additional 2 tablespoons (28g) to make it cohesive.

- Place the dough on a lightly floured work surface. Pat it into a rough rectangle about 3/4" thick. Fold it into thirds like a letter and roll gently with a floured rolling pin until the dough is 3/4" thick again.

- Cut the dough into circles with a biscuit cutter for traditional round biscuits; a 2 3/8" cutter makes nice-sized biscuits. Or to avoid leftover dough scraps, cut the dough into squares or diamonds with a bench knife or sharp knife.

- Place the biscuits bottom side up on your prepared baking sheet; turning them over like this yields biscuits with nice, smooth tops. Brush the biscuits with milk, to enhance browning.

- Bake the biscuits for 15 to 20 minutes, until they're lightly browned. Remove them from the oven, and serve warm.

- Store any leftover biscuits, well wrapped, at room temperature for several days. Freeze for longer storage. Biscuits are always best when they're rewarmed before serving.

## NUTRITION FACTS

Per Serving: 66 calories; 2.9 g total fat; 1 mg cholesterol; 127 mg sodium. 8.4 g carbohydrates; 1.3 g protein;

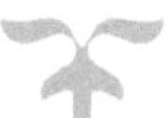

## COTTAGE CHEESE PANCAKES

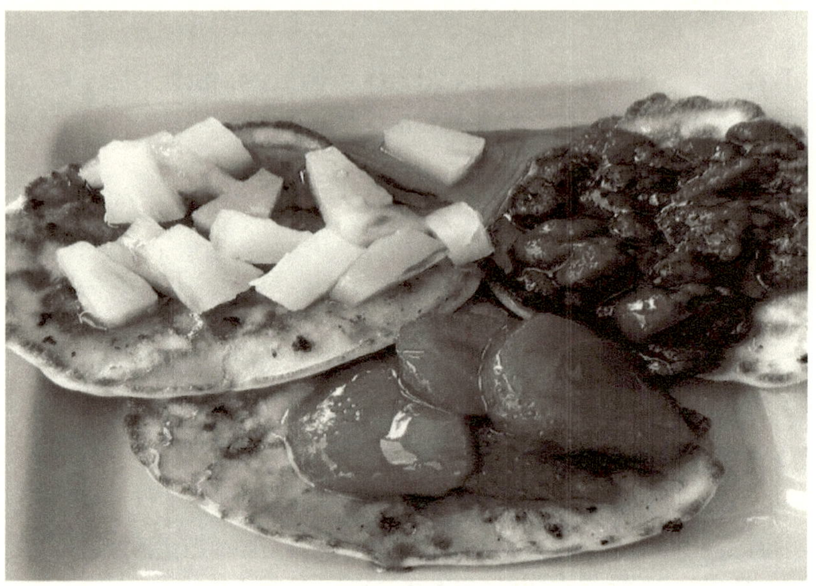

Cottage cheese is a great ingredient that is rich in calcium, protein, and various vitamins. If you are looking for cottage cheese recipes that are healthy, you've come to the right place.

These pancakes keep their springy quality with the help of the eggs. But the springiness also comes from whizzing the mixture together in your blender (or stick blender), whichs adds a bit of air to the batter.

# INGREDIENTS

- 1/2 cup old-fashioned oats
- 1/2 cup cottage cheese
- 2 large eggs
- 1/8 teaspoon kosher salt
- Maple syrup, jam, or sliced berries, for serving

# DIRECTIONS

Prep
10 m

Cook
10 m

Ready In
1 hr 30 m

Servings
3

- Place the oats, cottage cheese, eggs, and salt in a blender and process on high speed until well-combined, about 30 seconds.
- Heat a large nonstick frying pan over medium heat. Working in batches, add the batter in 2-tablespoon portions, spacing them evenly apart. Cook until the

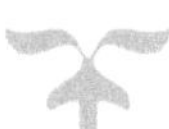

pancakes are set around the edges and deep golden-brown on the bottom, 2 to 3 minutes (this batter won't bubble up like traditional pancake batter). Gently flip the pancakes with a thin spatula and cook until the second side is golden-brown, 1 to 2 minutes more. Transfer to a plate.

- Repeat cooking the remaining batter. These pancakes are best when eaten fresh off the griddle and still warm. Serve with maple syrup, honey, or jam.

## NUTRITION FACTS

Per Serving:273 calories; 17.5 g total fat; 221 mg cholesterol; 632 mg sodium. 12.1 g carbohydrates; 16.9 g protein;

# INDIVIDUAL BAKED EGGS

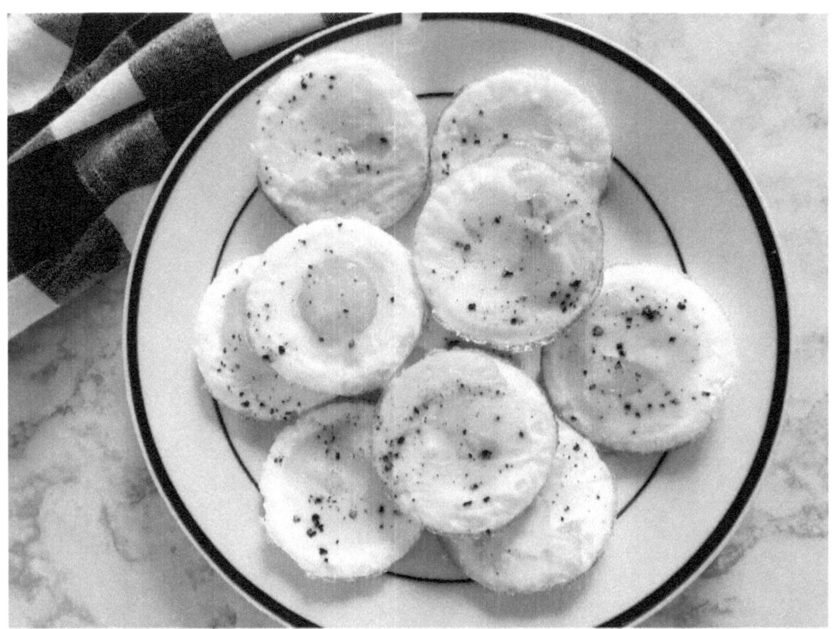

A very easy idea with a minimum of fuss or muss for any number of people. Individual Baked Eggs surrounded by a strip of bacon, and topped with a square of cheese. These eggs take on a very pleasing flavor just by baking instead of cooking them in the more conventional manner. Great not having splatters all over, and being able to do 12 or more eggs at one time.

# INGREDIENTS

- 1 slice bacon
- 1 teaspoon melted butter
- 1 egg
- ¼ slice Cheddar cheese

# DIRECTIONS

Prep
10 m

Cook
20 m

Ready In
30 m

Servings
1

- Preheat oven to 350 degrees F (175 degrees C).

- Place bacon in a large, deep skillet. Cook over medium high heat until evenly brown, but still flexible. Wrap bacon slice around the inside of a muffin cup. Place a teaspoon of butter (or bacon grease) in the bottom of muffin cup. Drop in egg.

- Bake in preheated oven for 10 to 15 minutes. Place 1/4 slice of cheese over egg, and continue cooking until cheese is melted and egg is cooked.

## NUTRITION FACTS

Per Serving:174 calories; 14.3 g total fat; 212 mg cholesterol; 305 mg sodium. 0.6 g carbohydrates; 10.7 g protein;

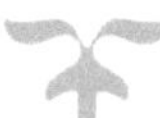

# OVEN BAKED OMELET

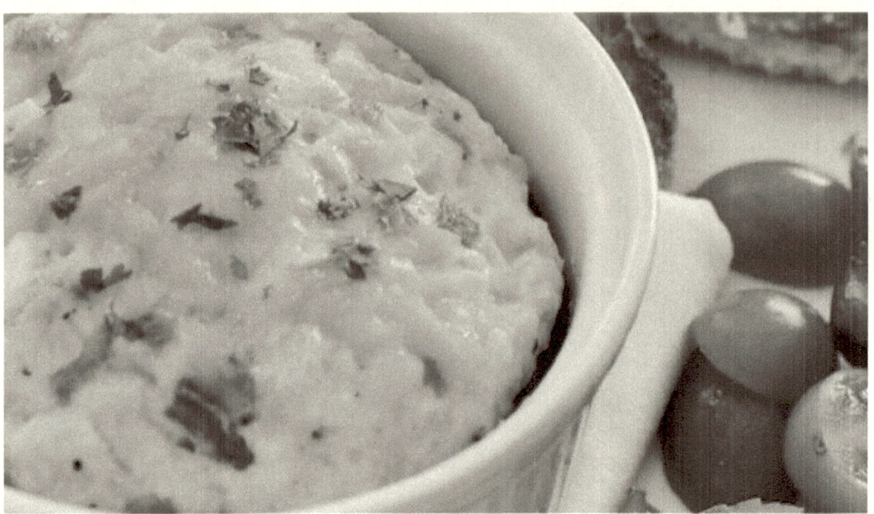

Love the taste of eggs, but don't love standing over the stove to flip, stir, or babysit them as they cook? Introducing the Baked Western Omelet, which is an easy and healthy way to serve eggs to a crowd! Perfect for breakfast, brunch, lunch or dinner!

# INGREDIENTS

- 8 large eggs
- 1/2 cup half-and-half cream
- 1 cup shredded cheddar cheese
- 1 cup finely chopped fully cooked ham
- 1/4 cup finely chopped green pepper
- 1/4 cup finely chopped onion

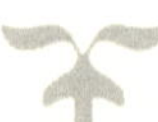

# DIRECTIONS

Prep
10 m

Cook
30 m

Ready In
40 m

Servings
4

- Preheat oven to 350 degrees F (175 degrees C). Grease an 8x8-inch baking dish with butter.
- Beat eggs, sour cream, milk, and salt in a bowl until blended. Stir in green onions. Pour mixture in the prepared baking dish.
- Bake in the preheated oven until set, 25 to 30 minutes. Sprinkle Cheddar cheese over eggs and continue baking until cheese is melted, 2 to 3 minutes more.

# NUTRITION FACTS

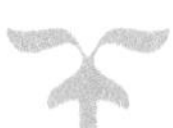

Per Serving: 185 calories; 14.1 g fat; 2.8 g carbohydrates; 12 g protein; 296 mg cholesterol; 546 mg sodium.

# DUTCH BABIES

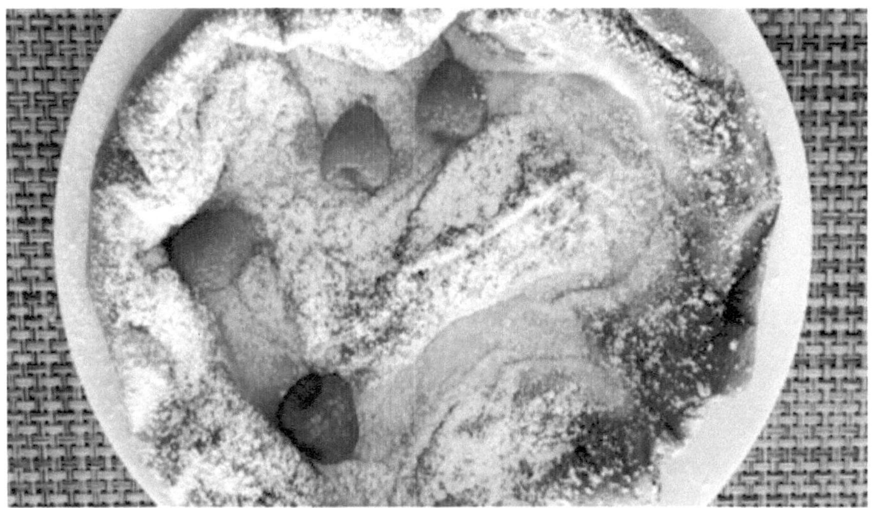

This large, fluffy pancake is excellent for breakfast, brunch, lunch and dessert any time of year. And it comes together in about five blessed minutes. Just dump all of the ingredients into a blender, give it a good whirl, pour it into a heated skillet sizzling with butter, and pop it into the oven.

## INGREDIENTS

- 3 eggs
- ½ cup flour
- ½ cup milk
- 1 tablespoon sugar
- 4 tablespoons unsalted butter

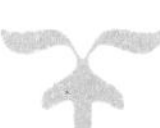

# DIRECTIONS

Prep
5 m

Cook
20 m

Ready In
25 m

Servings
4

- Preheat oven to 450 degrees F (230 degrees C). Lightly grease four 9 inch cake pans.
- In a large bowl, beat together cream, flour, salt and eggs. Pour into prepared pans.
- Bake in preheated oven until puffed and golden, about 15 to 20 minutes.

# NUTRITION FACTS

Per Serving: 212 calories; 16.7 g fat; 7.2 g carbohydrates; 8.5 g protein; 250 mg cholesterol; 236 mg sodium.

# HAM AND CHEESE OMELET CASSEROLE

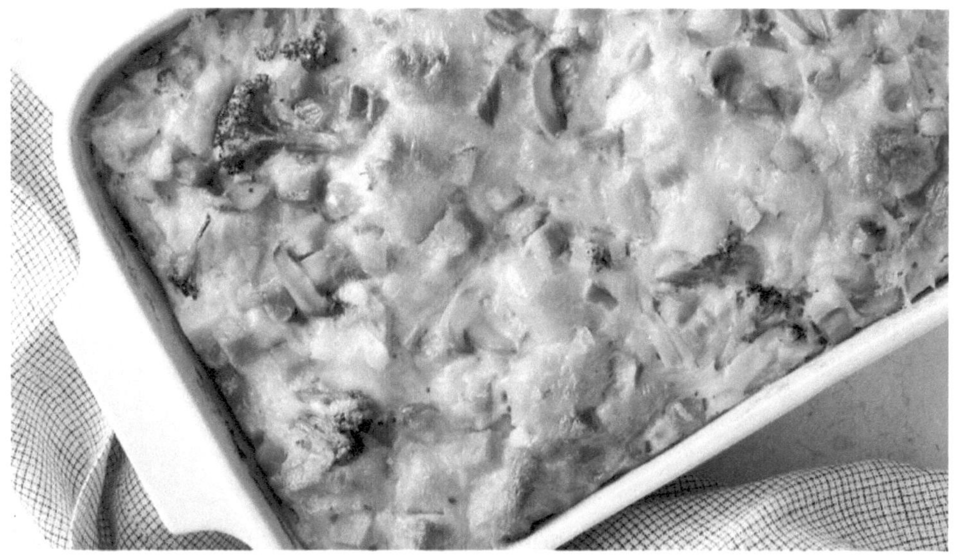

Delicious one dish meal. Breakfast for breakfast, for lunch or for dinner! Serve hot with hash browns if desired.

## INGREDIENTS

- 8 eggs
- 1 cup milk
- salt and pepper to taste
- 2 cups diced ham
- 1 cup shredded American cheese

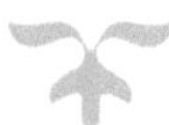

# DIRECTIONS

Prep
15 m

Cook
45 m

Ready In
1 h

Servings
4

- Preheat oven to 350 degrees F (175 degrees C).

- Beat eggs in a large bowl, making sure that they are mixed very well and have a 'frothy' top. Add the milk, salt and pepper. Mix well. Stir in ham, then add cheese pieces and stir well. Pour mixture into a well greased 4 quart casserole dish and bake in the preheated oven for 50 to 60 minutes or until top is lightly browned.

# NUTRITION FACTS

Per Serving: 407 calories; 27.9 g total fat; 443 mg cholesterol; 1440 mg sodium. 6.6 g carbohydrates; 31.7 g protein;

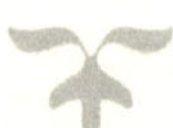

# OVEN SCRAMBLED EGGS

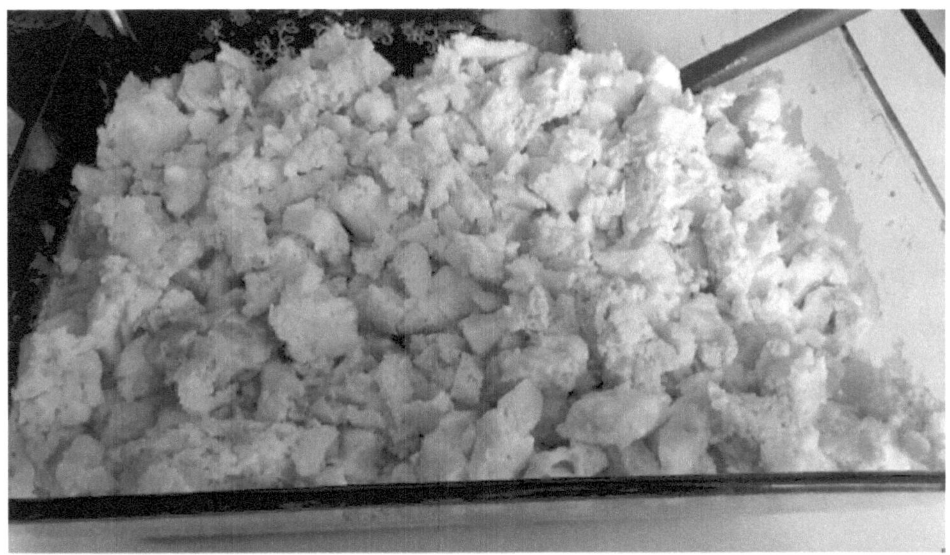

it's morning. Your stomach is growling. Your family is hungry for breakfast. Maybe you even have company over for brunch! Scrambled eggs seem like a good idea, but you don't want to slave over a hot stove all morning! Plus, who has a pan big enough to cook a DOZEN eggs on the stove top? Not me! Solution: Oven Baked Scrambled Eggs!

## INGREDIENTS

- 1/2 cup butter or margarine, melted
- 24 eggs
- 2 1/4 teaspoons salt

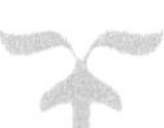

- 2 1/2 cups milk

# DIRECTIONS

Prep
10 m

Cook
25 m

Ready In
35 m

Servings
8

- Preheat the oven to 350 degrees F (175 degrees C).
- Pour melted butter into a glass 9x13 inch baking dish. In a large bowl, whisk together eggs and salt until well blended. Gradually whisk in milk. Pour egg mixture into the baking dish.
- Bake uncovered for 10 minutes, then stir, and bake an additional 10 to 15 minutes, or until eggs are set. Serve immediately.

# NUTRITION FACTS

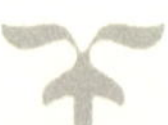

Per Serving: 236 calories; 18.6 g fat; 3.2 g carbohydrates; 14.3 g protein; 396 mg cholesterol; 651 mg sodium.

# MOCK OATMEAL

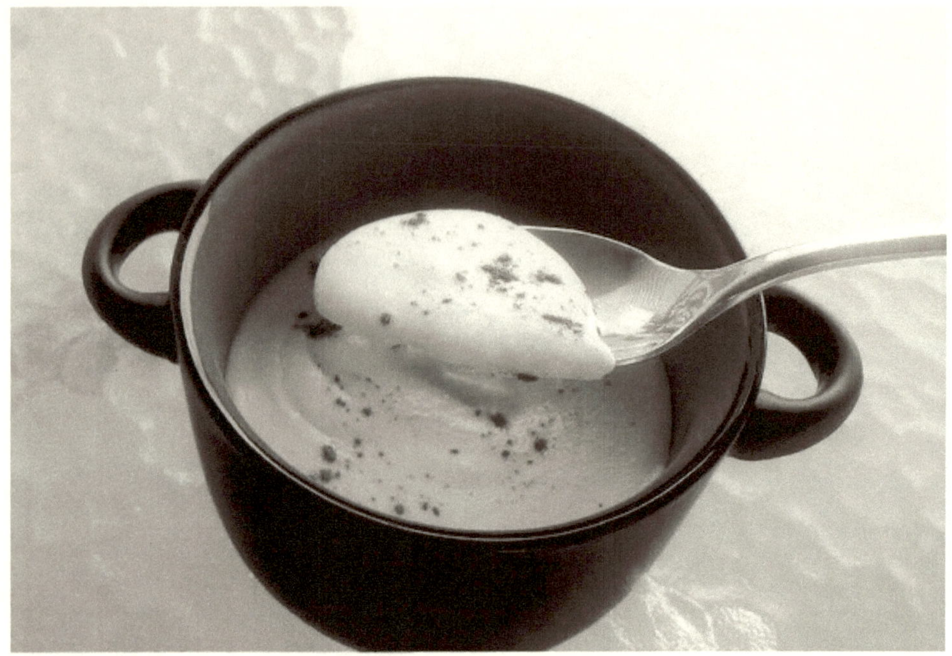

This is a warm and satisfying way to start the day - a nice change from bacon and eggs when you are on a low-carb diet. It may sound odd, but give it at try - it's actually yummy. This can also be made using maple extract.

## INGREDIENTS

- ½ cup ricotta cheese
- 1 tablespoon granular sucrolose sweetener

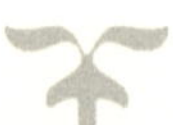

- 1 teaspoon vanilla extract

# DIRECTIONS

Prep
2 m

Cook
3 m

Ready In
5 m

Servings
1

- In a cereal bowl, stir together the ricotta cheese, sweetener and vanilla. Cover with plastic wrap, and poke a hole to vent steam. Heat in the microwave oven for 2 to 3 minutes, until hot. Remove plastic wrap, stir and enjoy.

## NUTRITION FACTS

Per Serving: 12 calories; 0 g total fat; 0 mg cholesterol; 0 mg sodium. 0.5 g carbohydrates; 0 g protein;

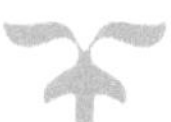

# EGG FLIPPED OVER

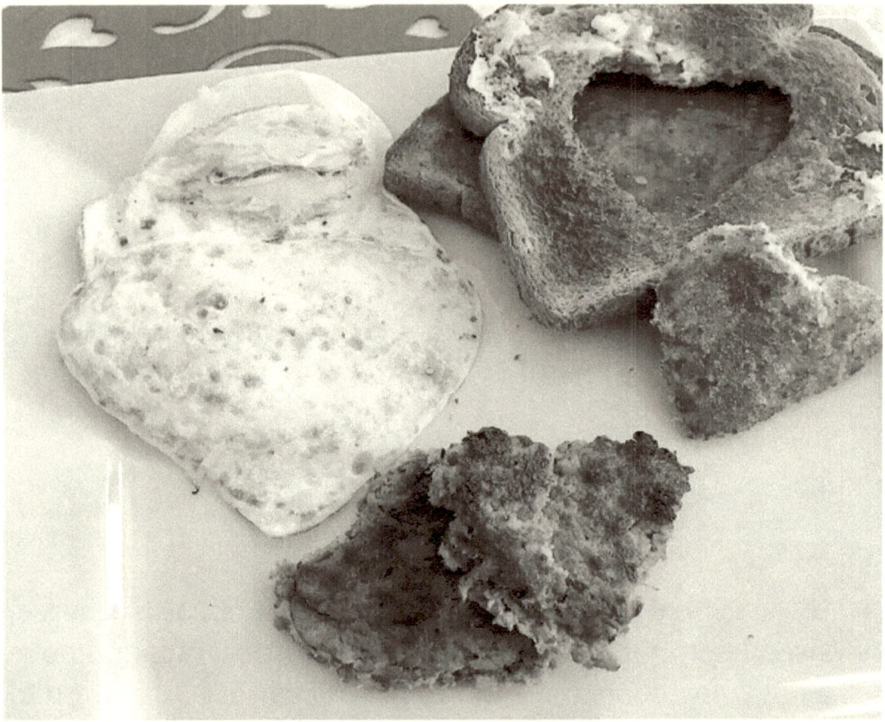

This recipe is easy, fun and good for kids.

## INGREDIENTS

- 1 teaspoon butter
- 1 egg
- 2 tablespoons milk
- 1 slice Cheddar cheese

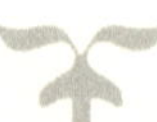

# DIRECTIONS

Prep
5 m

Cook
3 m

Ready In
8 m

Servings
1

- Melt butter in a small skillet over medium heat. In a small bowl, whisk together egg and milk; pour into skillet. Cook until bubbles appear, then flip over. Cover with cheese. Cook 10 seconds, or until cheese is melted.

# NUTRITION FACTS

Per Serving: 237 calories; 19 g total fat; 229 mg cholesterol; 287 mg sodium. 2.2 g carbohydrates; 14.4 g protein;

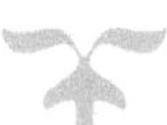

# HEART ATTACK EGGS

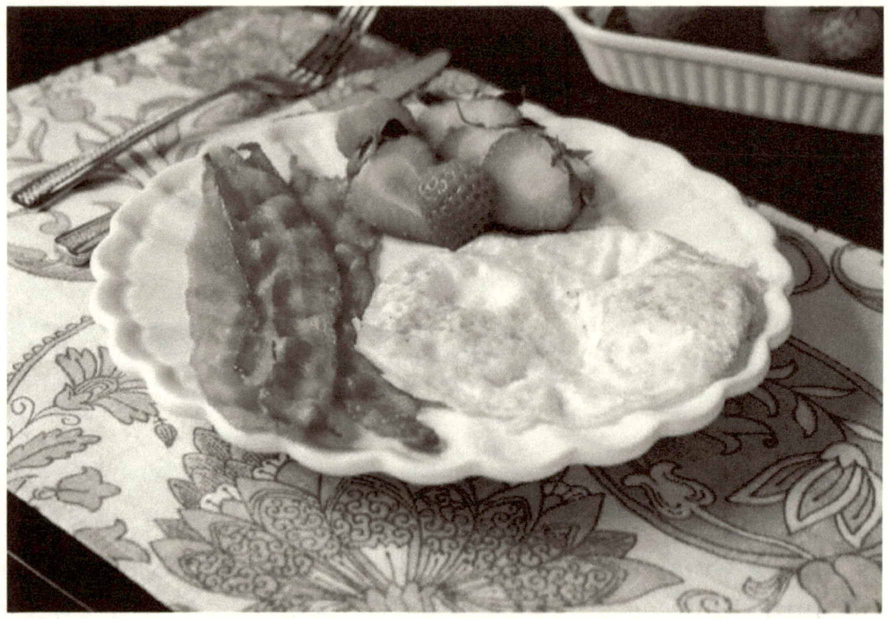

This is a great breakfast, especially on the weekend. You fry bacon on a skillet, then after the bacon is crispy, fry eggs in the bacon grease. Garnish your plate with toast or fruit.

## INGREDIENTS

- 6 slices bacon
- 3 eggs
- salt and pepper to taste

# DIRECTIONS

Prep
2 m

Cook
30 m

Ready In
32 m

Servings
1

- Fry the bacon in a large skillet over medium heat until crisp. Remove from the pan, and set on paper towels to drain. Crack the eggs into the pan with the bacon grease so that they are about 1 inch apart. Season with salt and pepper. When the eggs look firm, flip them over, and cook on the other side to your desired doneness. Transfer to a plate and serve with bacon.

## NUTRITION FACTS

328 calories; 30.2 g total fat; 224 mg cholesterol; 536 mg sodium. 0.8 g carbohydrates; 12.8 g protein;

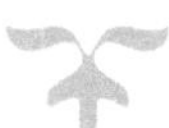

# SPAM AND EGGS

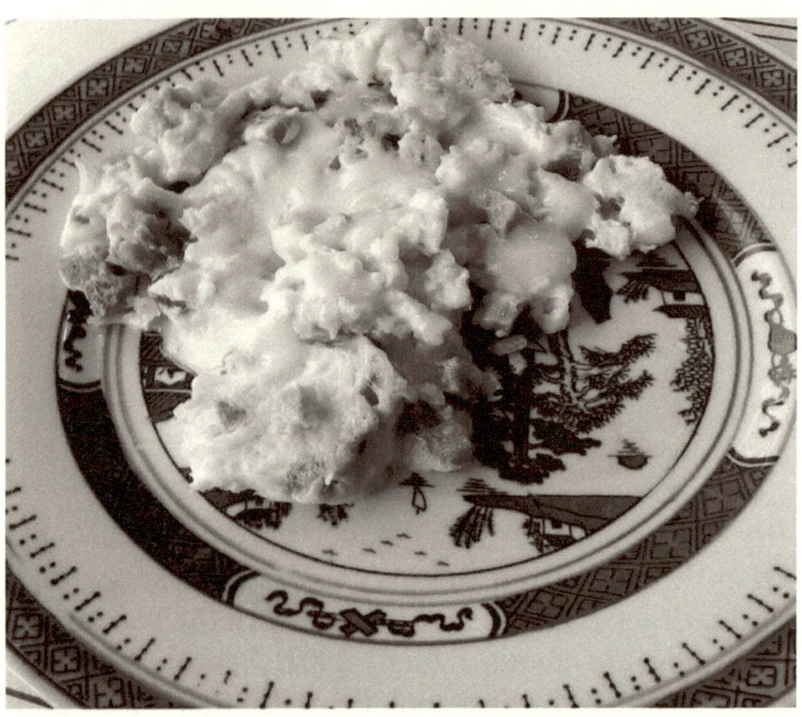

I'm on a diet where I have to eat over twice as much protein as carbohydrates. This was hard for a rice and biscuits lover such as myself. After days of eating tuna and eggs (not together), I came up with this recipe. It's quick and tasty.

# INGREDIENTS

- 1 (12 ounce) container fully cooked luncheon meat (e.g. Spam), cubed
- 2 eggs, beaten
- 2 ounces Cheddar cheese, grated

# DIRECTIONS

Prep
5 m

Cook
10 m

Ready In
15 m

Servings
1

- Heat a non-stick skillet over medium heat. Pour in eggs, then Spam. Cook, stirring, until eggs are nearly done, then sprinkle cheese over, and stir until melted.

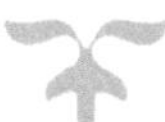

# NUTRITION FACTS

707 calories; 60.1 g total fat; 333 mg cholesterol; 2546 mg sodium. 5.8 g carbohydrates; 35.6 g protein;

# CHEESY HORSERADISH OMELET

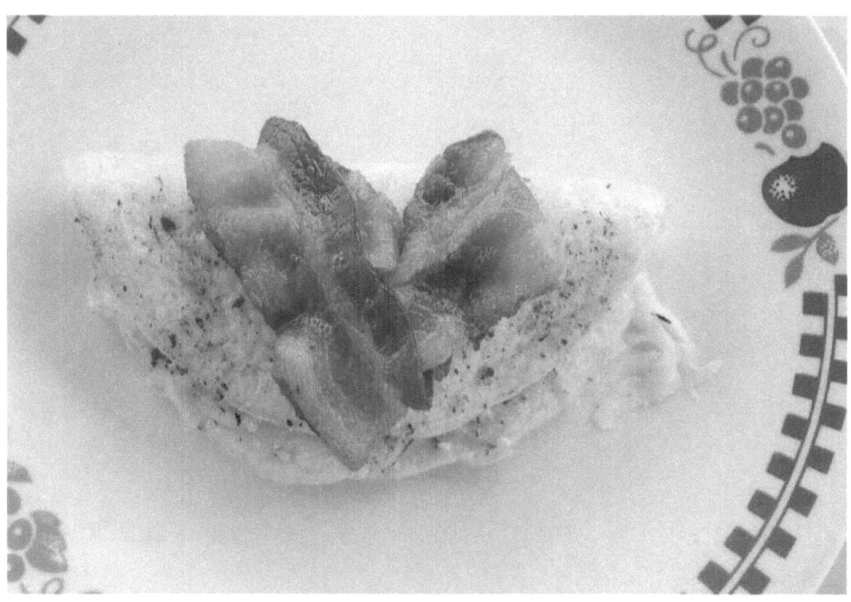

A tangy, ooey gooey omelet sure to please the pampered palette. I like to use Dubliner Irish cheese instead of Parmesan if I can get it.

## INGREDIENTS

- 2 eggs
- 1 ½ teaspoons prepared horseradish
- 1 teaspoon salt-free herb seasoning blend
- ½ cup shredded Cheddar cheese
- ¼ cup freshly grated Parmesan cheese

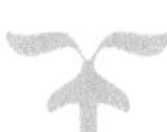

# DIRECTIONS

Prep
15 m

Cook
10 m

Ready In
35 m

Servings
1

- In a medium bowl, whisk together the eggs and herb seasoning blend.

- Place a lightly greased skillet over medium-high heat. When hot, pour the egg mixture in, and turn the skillet to coat evenly. Cook until almost done, then flip over. Spread the top with horseradish and sprinkle with Cheddar and Parmesan cheeses. Continue to cook until the bottom is no longer raw. Fold in half and transfer to a plate for serving.

# NUTRITION FACTS

506 calories; 38.1 g total fat; 358 mg cholesterol; 902 mg sodium. 4.8 g carbohydrates; 34.9 g protein;

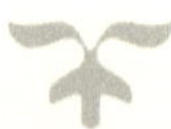

# PESTO SCRAMBLED EGGS

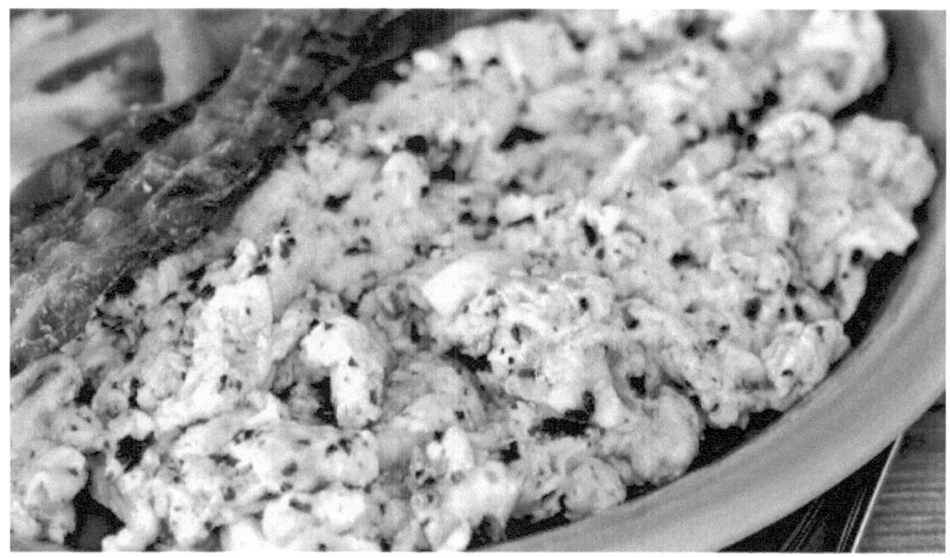

## INGREDIENTS

- 1 tablespoon vegetable oil
- 1 egg, lightly beaten
- 1/4 cup shredded Cheddar cheese
- salt and pepper to taste
- 1/2 teaspoon pesto

# DIRECTIONS

Prep
5 m

Cook
5 m

Ready In
10 m

Servings
1

- Heat oil in a skillet over medium heat. In a small bowl, combine egg, Cheddar cheese, salt and pepper. Pour into pan, and cook stirring for 3 to 5 minutes, or until desired doneness. Remove from heat, and stir in pesto.

# NUTRITION FACTS

Per Serving: 319 calories; 29.1 g fat; 0.9 g carbohydrates; 13.8 g protein; 216 mg cholesterol; 847 mg sodium.

## GROUND PORK OMELET

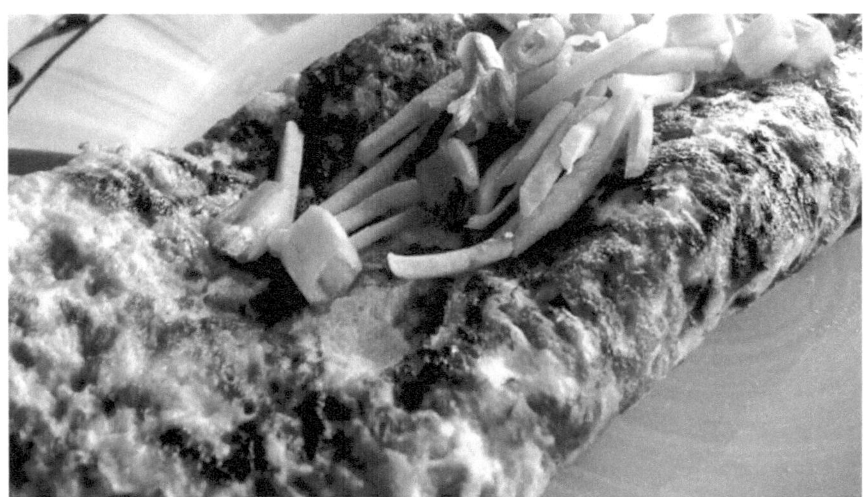

It smells good when it's cooked. Cut in wedges, and serve with jasmine rice. You can have it anytime! If you like spicy, put in some chile sauce.

# INGREDIENTS

- 2 tablespoons vegetable oil
- 3 eggs
- 2 ½ tablespoons fish sauce
- 1 pinch pepper
- 6 ounces ground pork

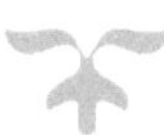

# DIRECTIONS

Prep
5 m

Cook
5 m

Ready In
10 m

Servings
2

- Heat oil in a wok or skillet over medium heat. In a medium bowl, whisk together eggs, fish sauce, pepper and ground pork. When oil is hot, pour in egg mixture. Fry until fully cooked, and golden on both sides.

# NUTRITION FACTS

Per Serving: 409 calories; 33.3 g total fat; 334 mg cholesterol; 1516 mg sodium. 1.5 g carbohydrates; 25.5 g protein;

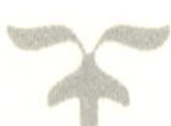

# HERBED CREAM CHEESE OMELET

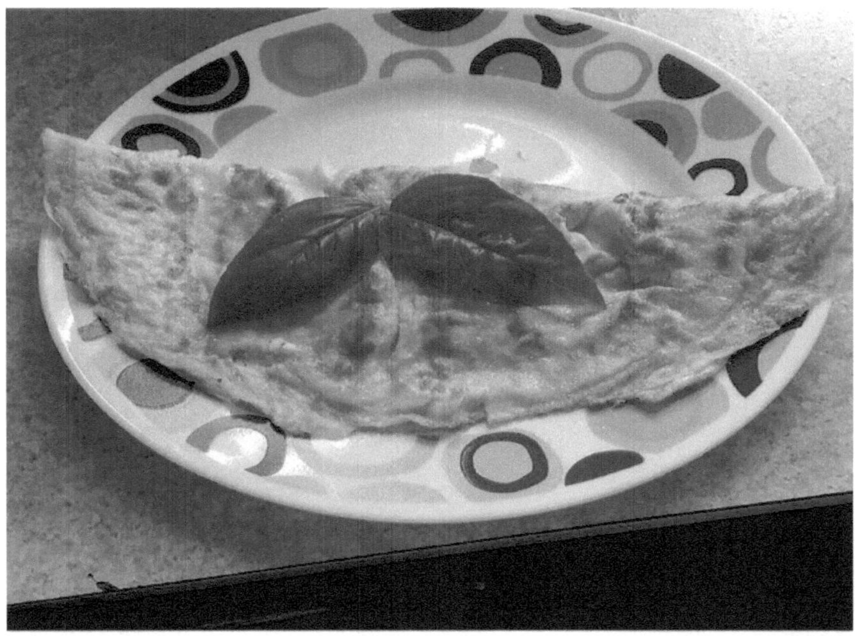

Somehow, when cream cheese is mixed with herbs and melted in an omelet, it acquires a wonderful taste that you wouldn't associate with cream cheese.
sauce.

## INGREDIENTS

- 4 ounces cream cheese, softened
- ½ cup fresh cilantro leaves
- salt and pepper to taste

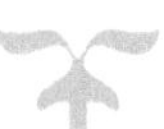

- 3 tablespoons butter
- 8 eggs

# DIRECTIONS

Prep
5 m

Cook
5 m

Ready In
10 m

Servings
4

- Mix the cream cheese with the cilantro in a bowl, adding salt and pepper to taste.

- Heat one-quarter of the butter in a well-seasoned omelet pan or 8 inch non-stick frying pan over medium-high heat. When the butter is hot and bubbling, swirl it around in the pan.

- Just before the butter begins to brown, beat 2 of the eggs and pour into pan. Lower the heat.

- After 10 seconds or so, the omelet will coagulate. Push the omelet to one side of the pan with a spoon or spatula, and let the raw egg run over the cleared skillet. Repeat this one more time, then take the skillet off the heat.

- Dab one quarter of the herbed cream cheese along the middle of the omelet from one side to the other. Season the omelet with additional salt and pepper to taste. If it has not completely set, place the pan over medium heat for a half minute longer. When the omelet is set, slide it from the pan onto a plate so that the omelet rolls up and the herbed cream cheese runs along the length of the roll. Serve it right away. Make three more omelets the same way, making sure the pan and butter get good and hot before adding the beaten eggs. Serve each one as soon as it is cooked.

## NUTRITION FACTS

Per Serving: 320 calories; 28.5 g total fat; 426 mg cholesterol; 288 mg sodium. 1.7 g carbohydrates; 14.9 g protein;

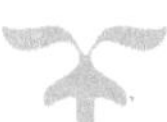

# BABY SPINACH OMELET

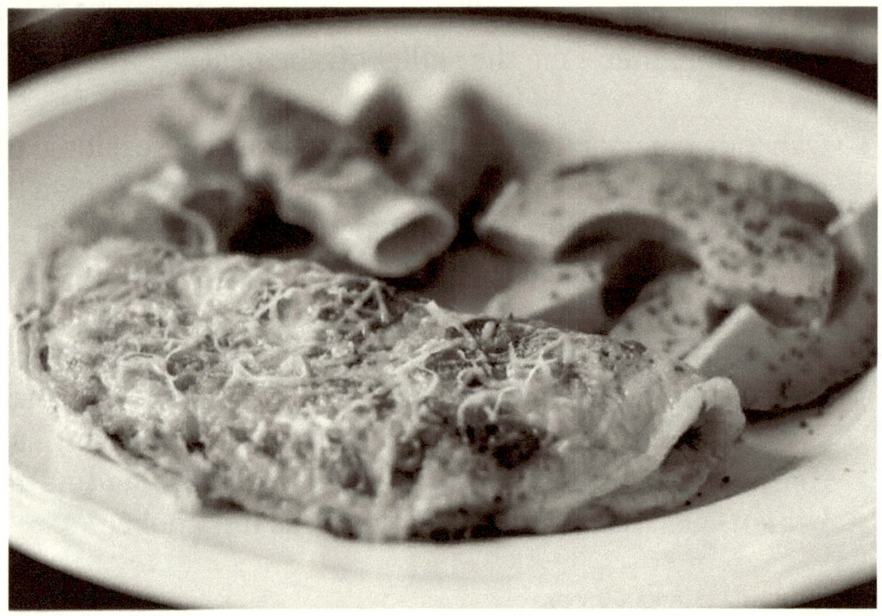

Tender baby spinach, Parmesan cheese, and a little nutmeg are cooked with eggs. A carb-cutter's perfect start for the day.

## INGREDIENTS

- 2 eggs
- 1 cup torn baby spinach leaves
- 1 ½ tablespoons grated Parmesan cheese
- ¼ teaspoon onion powder

- ⅛ teaspoon ground nutmeg
- salt and pepper to taste

# DIRECTIONS

Prep
6 m

Cook
9 m

Ready In
15 m

Servings
1

- In a bowl, beat the eggs, and stir in the baby spinach and Parmesan cheese. Season with onion powder, nutmeg, salt, and pepper.

- In a small skillet coated with cooking spray over medium heat, cook the egg mixture about 3 minutes, until partially set. Flip with a spatula, and continue cooking 2 to 3 minutes. Reduce heat to low, and continue cooking 2 to 3 minutes, or to desired doneness.

# NUTRITION FACTS

Per Serving: 186 calories; 12.3 g total fat; 379 mg cholesterol; 279 mg sodium. 2.8 g carbohydrates; 16.4 g protein;

## SAUSAGE, EGG, AND CHEESE SCRAMBLE

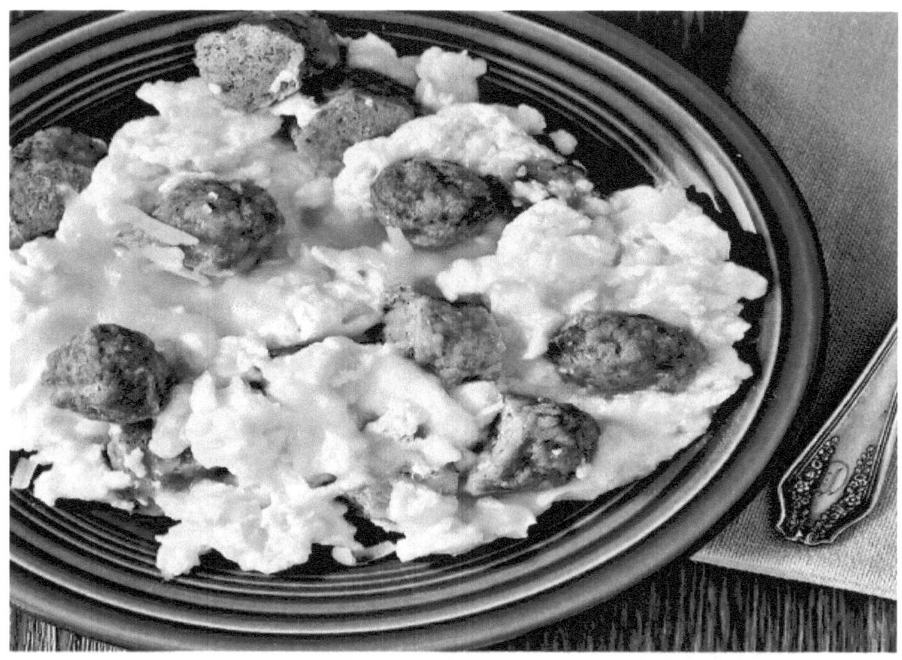

This is a tasty scramble of scrambled eggs, cheese, and pieces of sausage. Great for a Sunday morning family breakfast! You may use as much of whatever type of cheese you prefer for this recipe.

## INGREDIENTS

- 6 links pork sausage
- 6 eggs
- ¾ cup milk

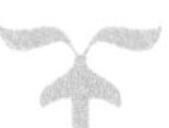

- ¾ cup shredded sharp Cheddar cheese

# DIRECTIONS

Prep
5 m

Cook
10 m

Ready In
15 m

Servings
2

- Place sausage in a large, deep skillet. Cook over medium high heat until evenly brown. Drain and chop into bite-size pieces; set aside.

- While sausage is cooking, beat eggs and milk together. Pour eggs into griddle. Add cheese and cook until eggs are set. Stir in sausage and serve warm.

# NUTRITION FACTS

Per Serving: 313 calories; 23.2 g total fat; 336 mg cholesterol; 468 mg sodium. 3 g carbohydrates; 22.5 g protein;

## EASY CLOUD BREAD

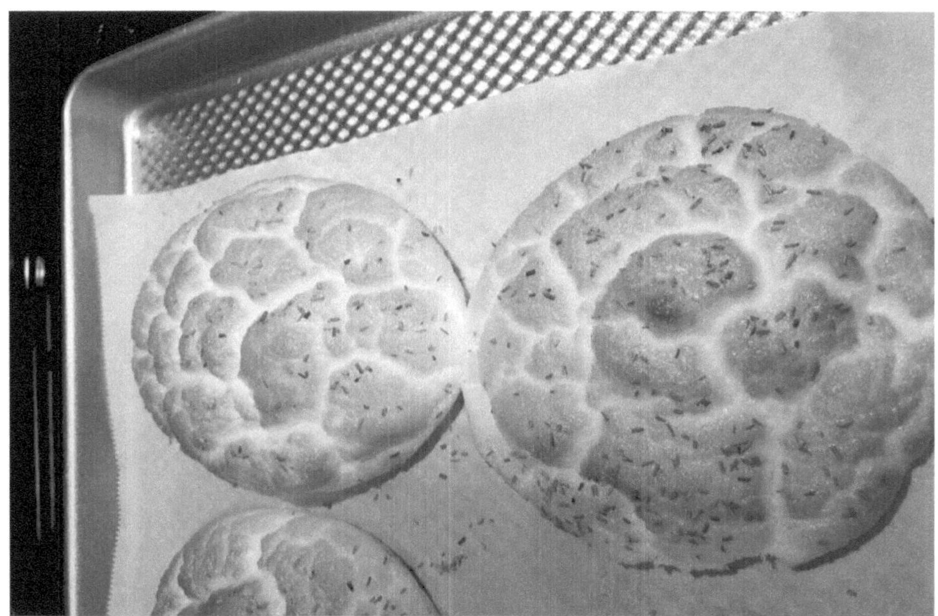

Cloud bread is soft and fluffy - like a cloud! It's a great substitute for 'regular' bread and is low in carbs. Although it's not firm enough to replace bread in a regular sandwich, I like to top one 'slice' with peanut butter and bananas, toast it with jam or with my favorite lunch meat and fillings!

## INGREDIENTS

- 3 large eggs, separated
- ¼ teaspoon cream of tartar
- 2 ounces cream cheese, very soft

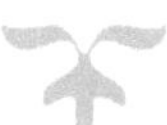

- 1 tablespoon white sugar

# DIRECTIONS

Prep
10 m

Cook
30 m

Ready In
40 m

Servings
2

- Preheat oven to 350 degrees F (175 degrees C). Line a baking sheet with parchment paper.

- Beat egg whites and cream of tartar together in a bowl until stiff peaks form.

- Mix egg yolks, cream cheese, and sugar together in a separate bowl using a wooden spoon and then mixing with a hand-held egg beater until mixture is very smooth and has no visible cream cheese. Gently fold egg whites into cream cheese mixture, taking care not to deflate the egg whites.

- Carefully scoop mixture onto the prepared baking sheet, forming 5 to 6 "buns".

- Bake in the preheated oven until cloud bread is lightly browned, about 30 minutes.

## NUTRITION FACTS

Per Serving: 93 calories; 6.9 g total fat; 124 mg cholesterol; 76 mg sodium. 3.1 g carbohydrates; 4.6 g protein;

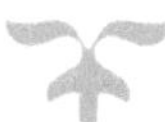

# VEGGIE POACHED EGGS

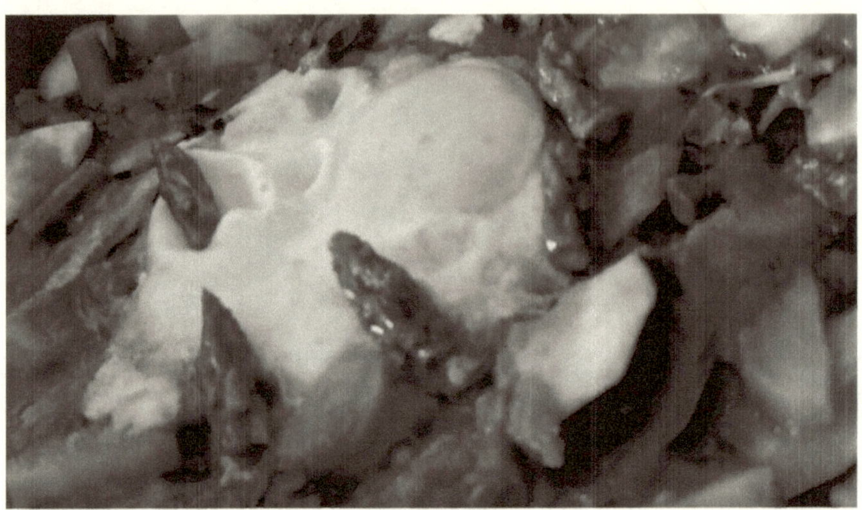

"Delicious and easy to make. A definite crowd pleaser, and there are many variations by using different vegetables, including broccoli, cauliflower and mushrooms. Season with your choice of spices."

## INGREDIENTS

- 1 1/2 tablespoons olive oil
- 1 cup fresh asparagus, trimmed and coarsely chopped
- 1 cup carrots, julienned
- 1/4 cup spaghetti sauce
- 4 eggs
- salt and pepper to taste

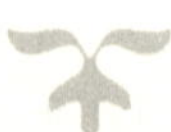

# DIRECTIONS

Prep
15 m

Cook
20 m

Ready In
35 m

Servings
2

- In a large frying pan, heat the oil over medium high heat. Add the asparagus, carrots and spaghetti sauce; cook on medium high heat until vegetables are soft. You may add a little water if necessary.
- Push the vegetables to the side of the pan to create four spaces for the eggs. Crack eggs directly into the holes, being careful not to break the yolk. Cook until eggs are done, but the yolk is still soft. Season with salt and pepper to taste. Remove from heat and serve immediately.

## NUTRITION FACTS

Per Serving: 147 calories; 10.6 g fat; 6.2 g carbohydrates; 7.5 g protein; 186 mg cholesterol; 294 mg sodium.

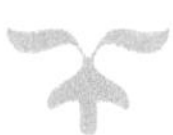

# HAM AND CHEESE CHOP CHOP

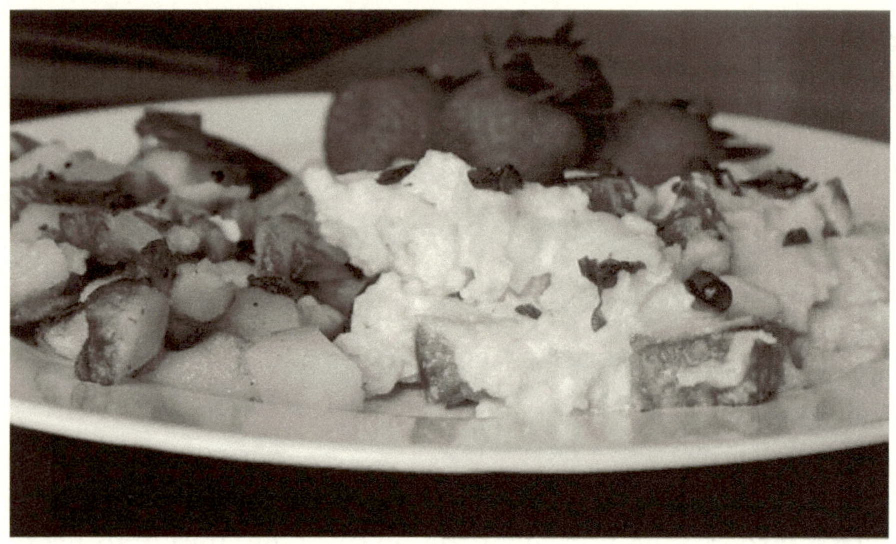

This is a great way to use up some Easter ham on the morning after. It's an easy-to-make omelet without all the fuss. Kids and adults both love it.

## INGREDIENTS

- 6 eggs
- 1 tablespoon milk
- 1 ½ cups cubed smoked ham
- ¾ cup shredded Cheddar cheese

# DIRECTIONS

Prep
5 m

Cook
5 m

Ready In
10 m

Servings
3

- Preheat a skillet over medium heat. Combine eggs and milk in a large bowl; beat well.

- Add ham to preheated skillet and warm until juicy. Add eggs and stir regularly until they start to set. While eggs are still soft, add cheese. Cook until eggs are firm and cheese is melted. Season with salt and pepper to taste and serve.

# NUTRITION FACTS

Per Serving:324 calories; 24.3 g total fat; 331 mg cholesterol; 912 mg sodium. 1.1 g carbohydrates; 24.5 g protein;

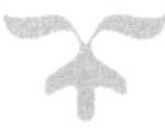

# EGG WHITE OMELET

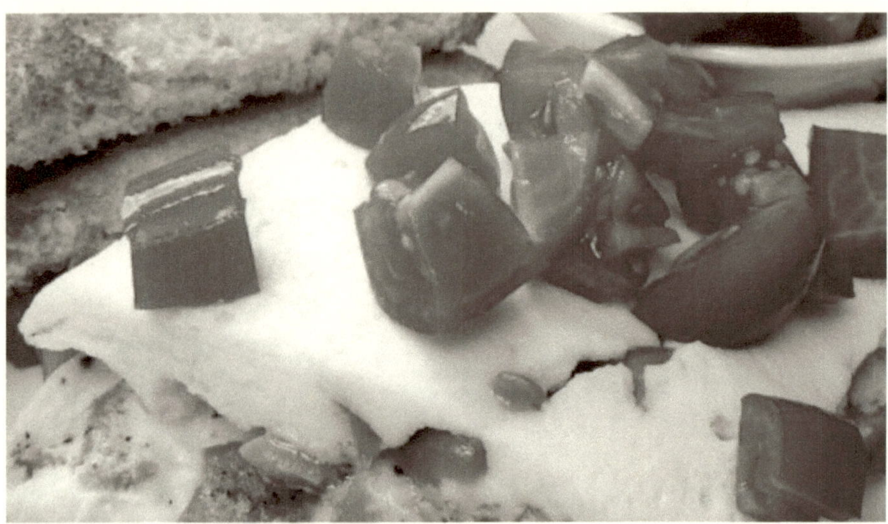

"This is a go-to breakfast every morning. Fast, easy, foolproof, customizable, and packed with protein, all for fewer calories than your average fast-food breakfast sandwich."

## INGREDIENTS

- cooking spray
- 2 tablespoons chopped onion
- 2 tablespoons chopped green bell pepper
- 2 tablespoons chopped mushrooms
- salt and ground black pepper to taste

- 1 (32 ounce) container refrigerated pasteurized egg white substitute

# DIRECTIONS

Prep
10 m

Cook
10 m

Ready In
20 m

Servings
4

- Spray a 9x5-inch glass or microwave-safe loaf pan with cooking spray; sprinkle the onion, green bell pepper, and mushrooms into the pan, and toss lightly with a fork just to mix. Season with salt and black pepper, and pour in the egg whites.
- Cook in a microwave oven on High setting for 3 minutes. Remove and stir the cooked egg white from the side of the pan into the rest of the ingredients; cook for 3 more minutes on High. If the omelet is still a little runny on top, slice it into chunks and turn them over in the loaf pan;

microwave for 30 more seconds on High. Adjust salt and pepper, and serve.

## NUTRITION FACTS

Per Serving: 128 calories; 0.1 g fat; 0.8 g carbohydrates; 24.9 g protein; 0 mg cholesterol; 371 mg sodium.

## CORNED BEEF HASH CAKES

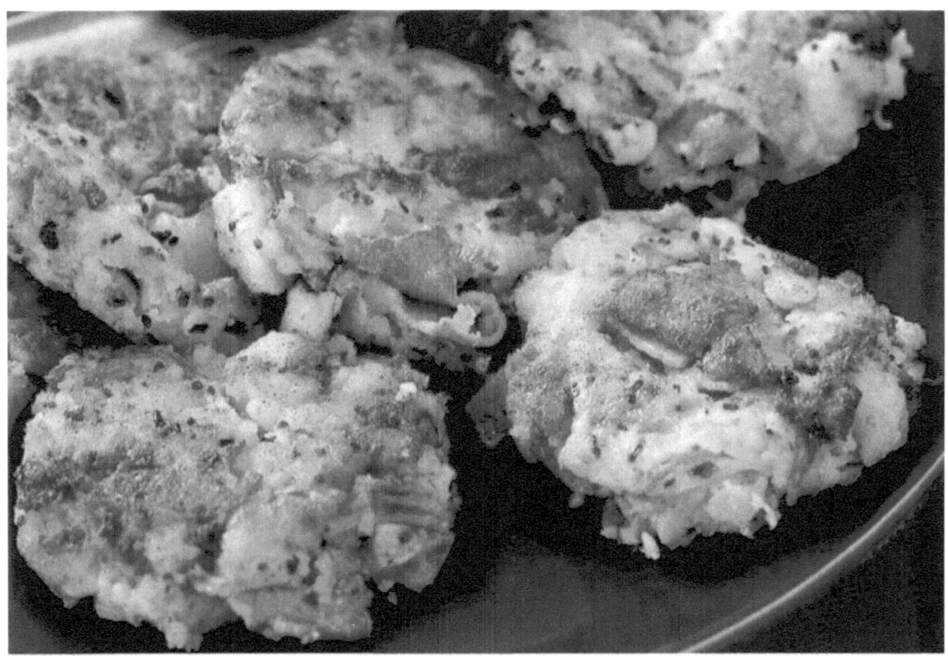

This recipe is delicious, quick and easy. It goes great with green beans, and is the perfect way to use left over mashed potatoes. Serve with green beans for a quick supper or eggs and toast for a hearty breakfast.

# INGREDIENTS

- 1 tablespoon vegetable oil
- 1 small onion, chopped
- 2 cups leftover mashed potatoes

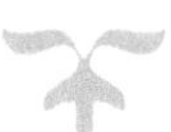

- salt and pepper to taste
- 1 cup shredded cooked corned beef

# DIRECTIONS

Prep
10 m

Cook
15 m

Ready In
25 m

Servings
2

- Heat oil in a large skillet over medium heat. Fry onion in oil until translucent. Transfer to a medium bowl, and mix with mashed potatoes and corned beef. Season with salt and pepper. Form into 8 patties. Fry patties in the skillet over medium-high heat until golden brown on both sides.

## NUTRITION FACTS

Per Serving: 114 calories; 6.1 g total fat; 13 mg cholesterol; 320 mg sodium. 9.7 g carbohydrates; 5 g protein;

# GREEN CHILI CASSEROLE

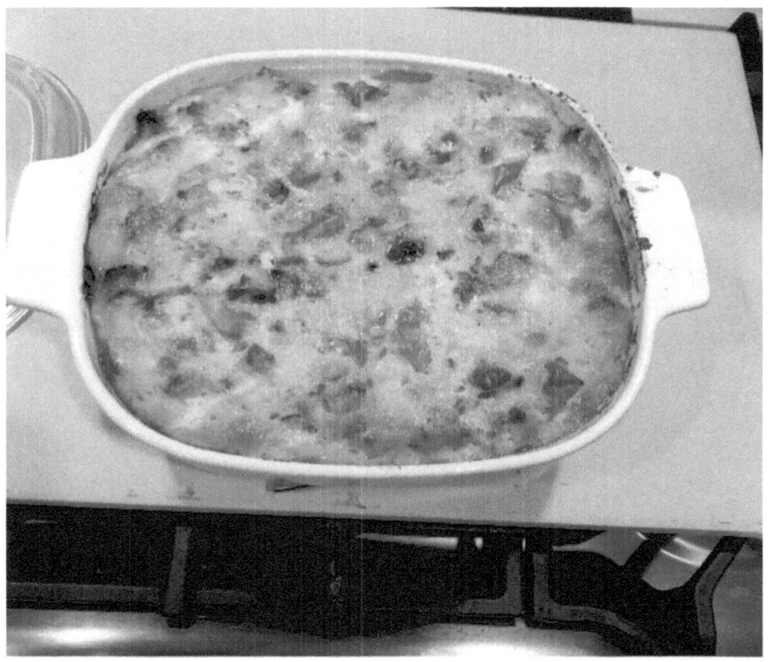

This casserole is also great when made with fresh long green chiles. Makes a wonderful brunch dish, but we also have it for lunch quite often.

## INGREDIENTS

- 2 (7 ounce) cans whole green chile peppers, drained
- 1 ½ cups shredded Cheddar cheese, divided
- ⅓ cup milk

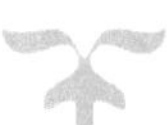

- 4 eggs, lightly beaten
- salt and pepper to taste

# DIRECTIONS

Prep
10 m

Cook
30 m

Ready In
40 m

Servings
8

- Preheat oven to 350 degrees F (175 degrees C). Grease an 8x12 inch baking dish.

- Line the bottom of dish with green chiles. Sprinkle with 1/2 cup shredded cheese. Repeat layers twice more. In a medium bowl, whisk together milk and eggs. Season with salt and pepper. Pour egg mixture over chiles and cheese.

- Bake in preheated oven for 25 to 30 minutes, or until filling is set. Let stand 5 to 10 minutes before serving.

# NUTRITION FACTS

Per Serving: 137 calories; 9.8 g total fat; 116 mg cholesterol; 746 mg sodium. 3.4 g carbohydrates; 9.2 g protein;

# LOW-CARB KETO BREAKFAST MUFFINS

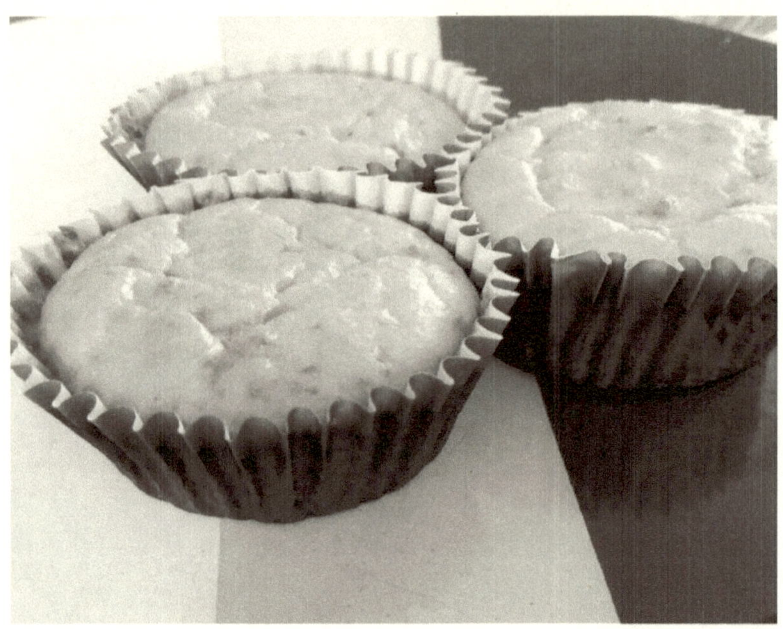

These keto muffins have only four ingredients, are low-carb, and keto-friendly. Amazingly delicious!

## INGREDIENTS

- 4 slices bacon, cooked and chopped
- 4 eggs
- ½ cup salsa
- ½ cup almond flour

# DIRECTIONS

Prep
10 m

Cook
30 m

Ready In
40 m

Servings
8

- Preheat the oven to 350 degrees F (175 degrees C). Grease 8 muffin cups with cooking spray.

- Blend bacon, eggs, salsa, and almond flour together in a blender on medium speed until thoroughly combined, about 30 seconds.

- Pour mixture into prepared muffin cups.

- Bake in the preheated oven until a toothpick inserted into the center of a muffin comes out clean, about 30 minutes. Let cool 10 minutes before serving.

# NUTRITION FACTS

Per Serving: 110 calories; 8.2 g total fat; 98 mg cholesterol; 236 mg sodium. 2.9 g carbohydrates; 6.7 g protein;

# VEGAN QUINOA OATMEAL

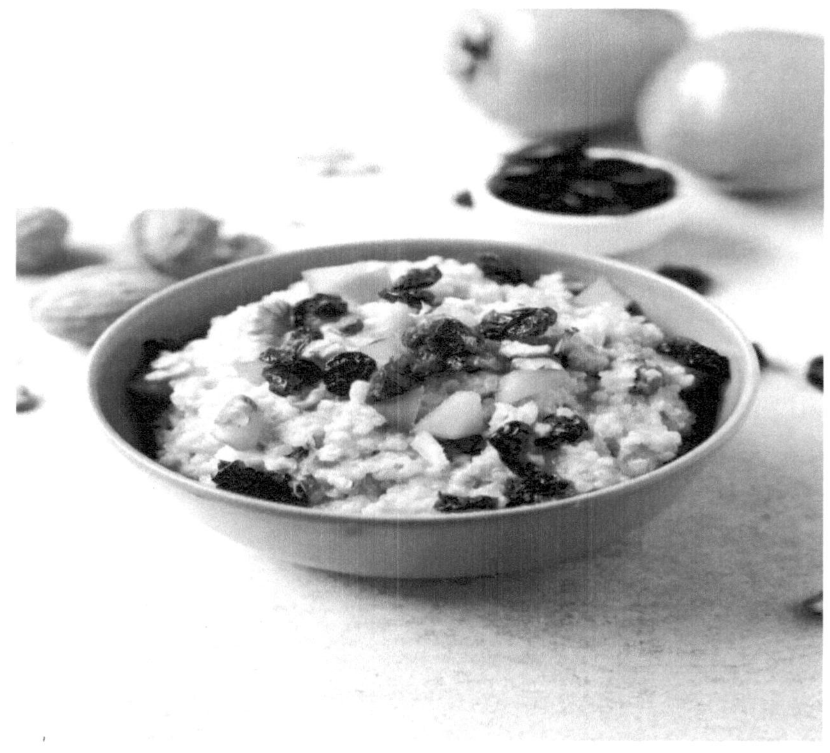

## INGREDIENTS

- 1/4 cup quinoa
- 1/4 cup rolled oats
- 2 tablespoons flaked coconut
- 2 tablespoons cacao nibs

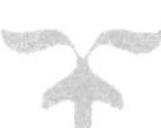

- 1 tablespoon molasses
- water to cover

## DIRECTIONS

Prep
5 m

Cook
15 m

Ready In
20 m

Servings
1

- Combine quinoa, oats, flaked coconut, cacao nibs, and molasses in a pot; cover with water. Bring to a boil and cover. Reduce heat and simmer until quinoa and oats are soft, 10 to 15 minutes. Add more water, 1 tablespoon at a time, if oatmeal becomes too dry.

## NUTRITION FACTS

Per Serving: 459 calories; 15.2 g fat; 71.8 g carbohydrates; 9.7 g protein; 0 mg cholesterol; 68 mg sodium.

# SPICY PORK SAUSAGE

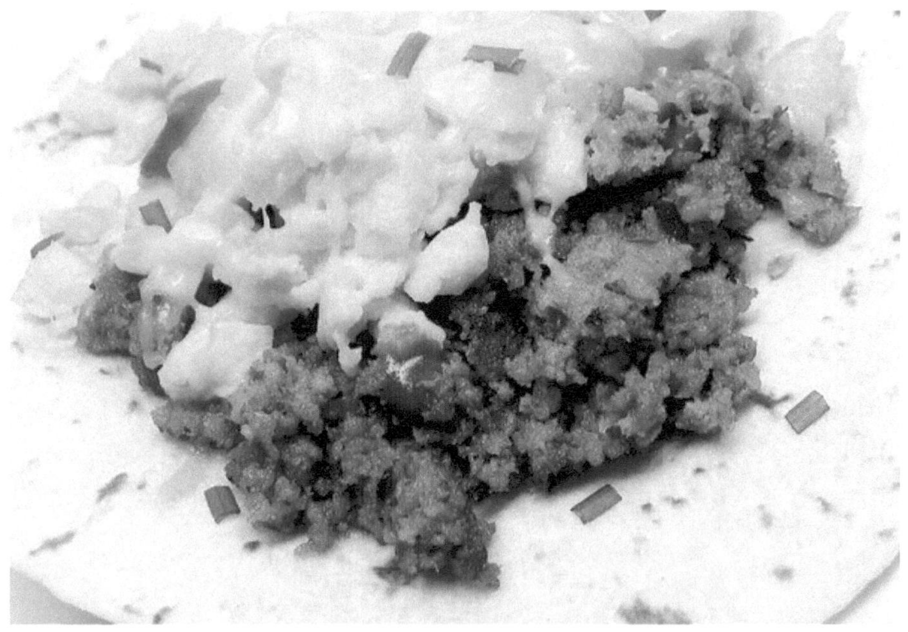

Jazz up any breakfast with these subtly spiced pork sausage. They're sure to perk up your taste buds and get your motor running!

## INGREDIENTS

- 1 pound fresh, ground pork sausage
- 1 tablespoon crushed red pepper
- 1 ½ tablespoons ground cumin

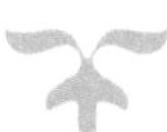

- 3 cloves garlic, finely chopped
- salt to taste

# DIRECTIONS

Prep
15 m

Cook
15 m

Ready In
30 m

Servings
4

- In a bowl, mix together with your hands Pork sausage, red pepper, cumin, garlic and salt. Form patties. Fry in a skillet over medium heat until well done.

# NUTRITION FACTS

Per Serving: 492 calories; 46.6 g total fat; 77 mg cholesterol; 762 mg sodium. 4.2 g carbohydrates; 14.1 g protein;

# SAUSAGE CHEESE BALLS

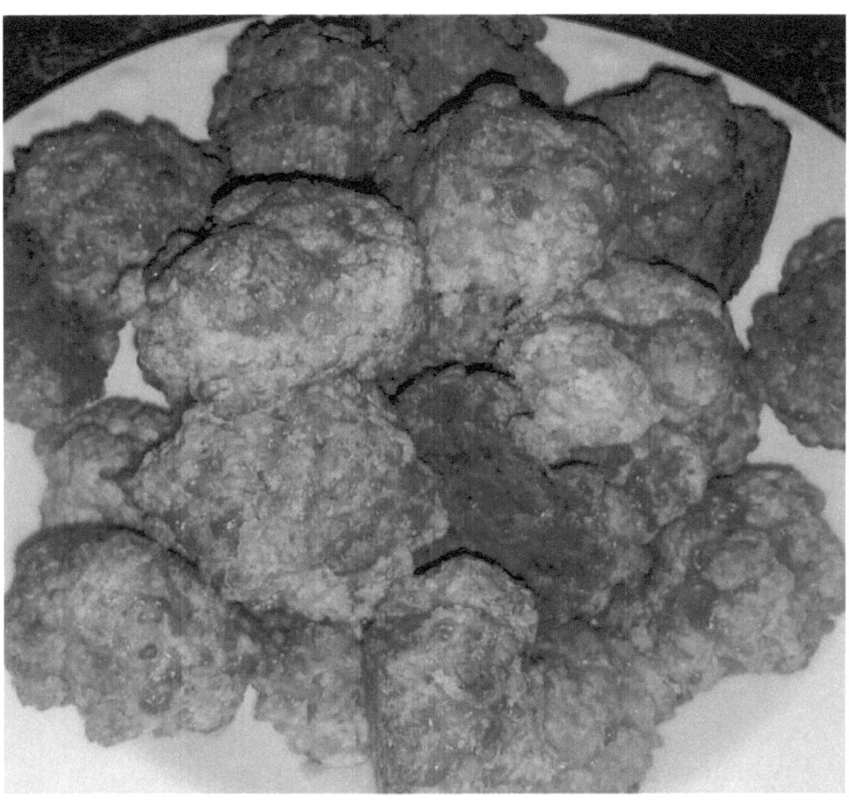

These are great for appetizers or for breakfast! Sausage cheese balls may be frozen before or after baking.

# INGREDIENTS

- 2 ounces sausage
- 1/4 cup and 2 tablespoons shredded Cheddar cheese
- 1/3 cup baking mix

# DIRECTIONS

Prep
10 m

Cook
15 m

Ready In
25 m

Servings
4

- Preheat oven to 400 degrees F (200 degrees C).

- In a medium bowl, combine the sausage, cheese, and dry baking mix. Mix together, and shape mixture into walnut-sized balls. Place on a foil-lined cookie sheet.

- Bake for 12 to 15 minutes. Serve hot.

# NUTRITION FACTS

Per Serving: 137 calories; 9.4 g total fat; 22 mg cholesterol; 354 mg sodium. 7.5 g carbohydrates; 5.5 g protein;

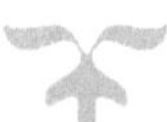

# LUNCH

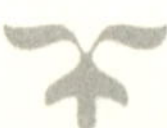

# CRAB SALAD

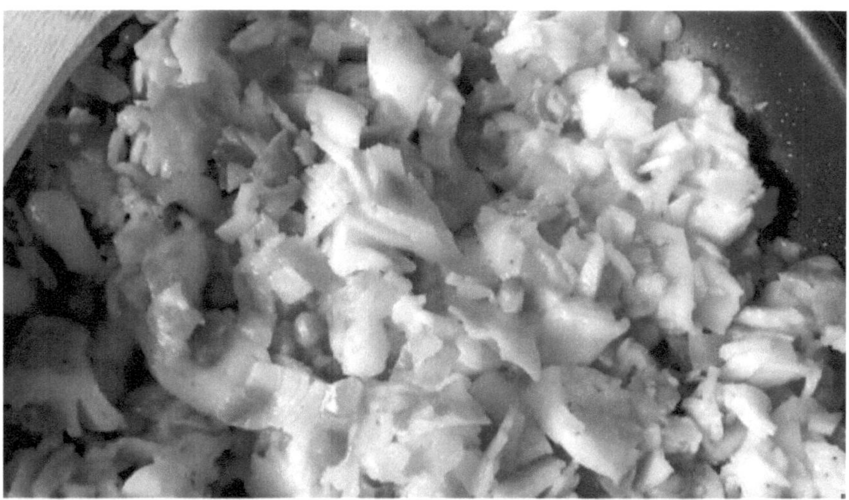

This crab salad is a blend of imitation crab, vegetables and herbs, all tossed in a simple creamy dressing. A quick and easy salad that's perfect served over lettuce, with crackers, or in a sandwich.

## INGREDIENTS

- 1/2 green bell pepper, chopped
- 1 onion, chopped
- 3 tablespoons butter
- 12 ounces imitation crabmeat
- 1 cup mayonnaise

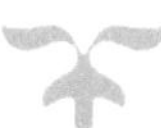

# DIRECTIONS

Prep
5 m

Cook
6 m

Ready In
11 m

Servings
4

- In a medium skillet, saute the green pepper and onion in the butter for 3 minutes, or until vegetables are tender.
- Stir in imitation crabmeat, and saute for another 3 minutes. Remove from heat, and put mixture into a medium bowl. Stir in mayonnaise. May be served warm or cold.

# NUTRITION FACTS

Per Serving: 283 calories; 26.4 g fat; 8.8 g carbohydrates; 3.7 g protein; 30 mg cholesterol; 541 mg sodium.

## HAM SPREAD

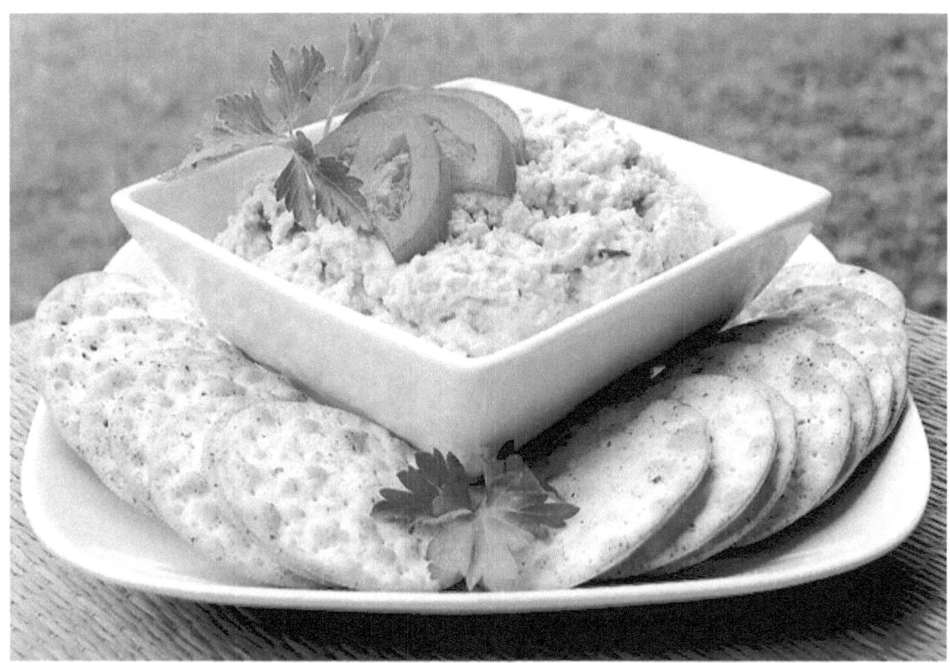

This recipe uses leftover ham with onion and dill pickle relish for a delicious sandwich spread or dip for crackers. You can substitute 10 green olives with pimentos for the dill pickle relish.

## INGREDIENTS

- 1 pound cooked ham
- ⅓ cup chopped onions
- 2 teaspoons dill pickle relish
- 1 teaspoon prepared mustard

- ¼ cup creamy salad dressing

# DIRECTIONS

Prep
15 m

Cook
0 m

Ready In
15 m

Servings
8

- Cut up ham to put into food processor, grind on pulse until very coarse. Add the onion and dill pickle relish close to the end of this stage. Put into mixing bowl and add mustard and creamy salad dressing; mix well.

## NUTRITION FACTS

Per Serving: 166 calories; 12.6 g total fat; 34 mg cholesterol; 810 mg sodium. 1.8 g carbohydrates; 10.6 g protein;

# HAM AND CHEESE SALAD

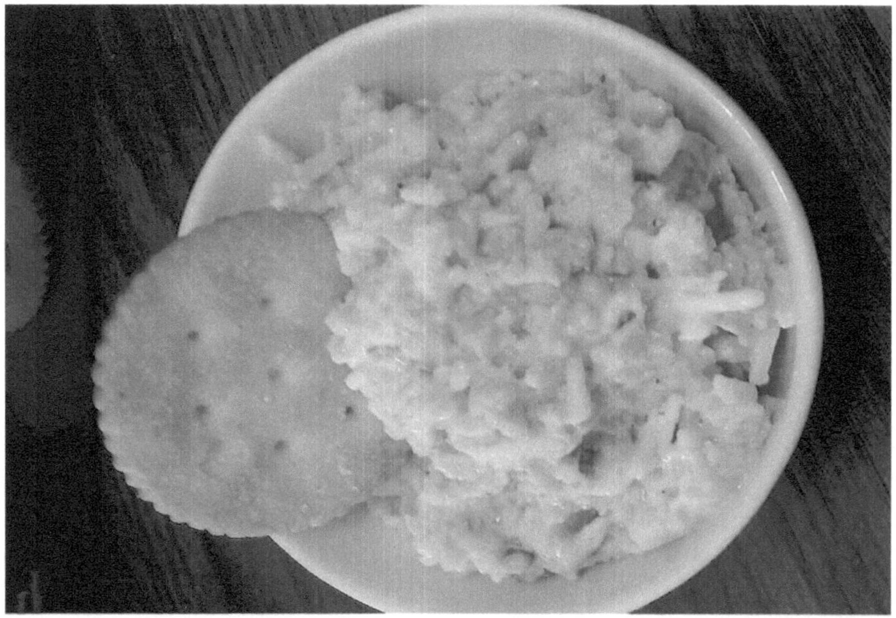

After making your own ham salad you'll never buy it prepared again. I first tried adding cheese to ham salad when I had to stretch a small amount of ham to make sandwiches for my children's lunches. It worked and they loved it!

## INGREDIENTS

- 2 cups chopped ham
- 1 cup shredded Cheddar cheese
- 2 stalks celery, chopped

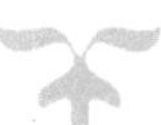

- ⅓ cup mayonnaise
- 1 ½ tablespoons prepared mustard

# DIRECTIONS

Prep
10 m

Cook
0 m

Ready In
10 m

Servings
5

- In a food processor, combine the ham and celery; pulse until finely chopped. Add cheese and pulse until mixed.

- Place mixture in a bowl and add the mayonnaise and mustard. Mix well; serve on sandwich or pita bread.

## NUTRITION FACTS

Per Serving: 284 calories; 24 g total fat; 56 mg cholesterol; 892 mg sodium. 3.4 g carbohydrates; 13.6 g protein;

# EGG SALAD

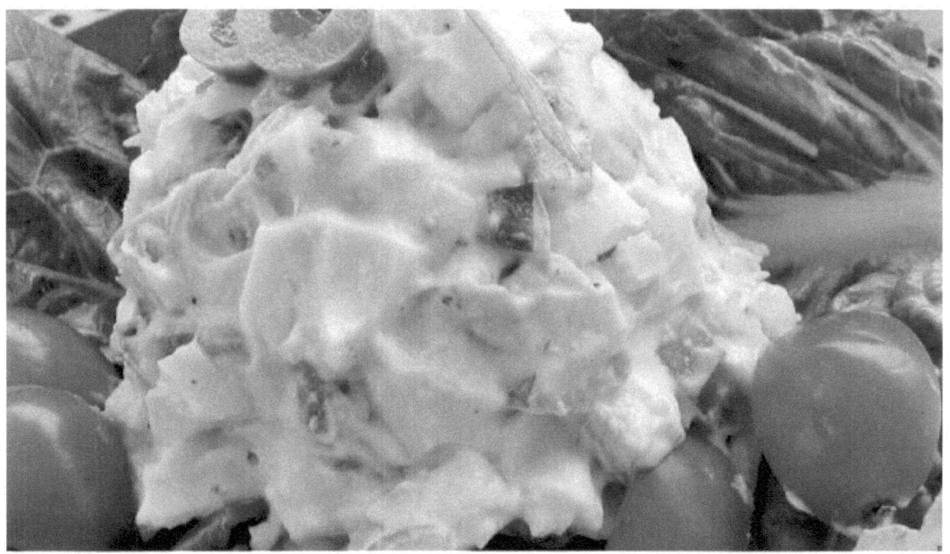

The key ingredient is the chopped pimento stuffed olives. Serve on toasted bread with lettuce and a bit of chopped celery."

Ingredients

- 8 eggs
- 1/2 cup mayonnaise
- 1 teaspoon ground black pepper
- 1/4 teaspoon paprika
- 2 tablespoons chopped pimento-stuffed green olives

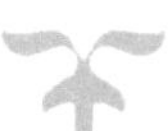

# DIRECTIONS

Prep
15 m

Cook
10 m

Ready In
25 m

Servings
4

- Place eggs in a medium saucepan with enough cold water to cover, and bring to a boil. Cover saucepan, remove from heat, and let eggs stand in hot water for 10 to 12 minutes. Remove from hot water, cool, peel, and chop.
- In a large bowl, mix eggs, mayonnaise, pepper, and paprika. Mash with a potato masher or fork until smooth. Gently stir in the olives. Refrigerate until serving.

## NUTRITION FACTS

Per Serving: 349 calories; 32.6 g fat; 2.2 g carbohydrates; 13 g protein; 382 mg cholesterol; 441 mg sodium.

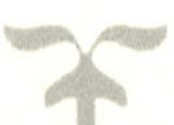

## FRESH LOBSTER SALAD

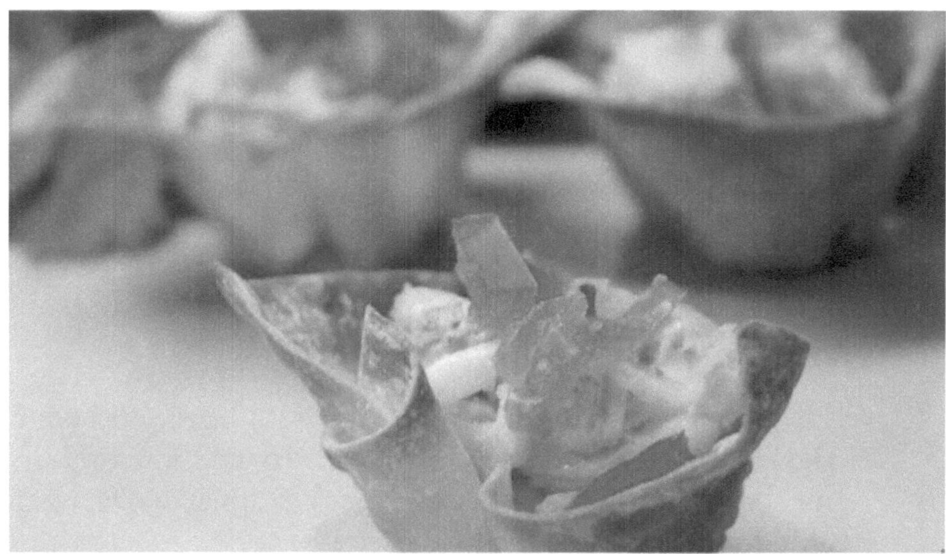

"A delicious treat anytime! A simple lobster salad with butter and just a hint of mayonnaise so that you can still taste the sweet lobster meat. Serve on toasted rolls or croissants. You won't be disappointed!"

## INGREDIENTS

- 1 pound cooked lobster meat, cut into bite-sized pieces
- 1/4 cup butter, melted
- 1/4 cup mayonnaise
- 1/8 teaspoon ground black pepper

# DIRECTIONS

Prep
10 m

Ready In
30 m

Servings
4

- Place the lobster chunks into a medium bowl, and pour the melted butter over. Toss to coat, then stir in mayonnaise and season with black pepper. Cover and chill for 20 minutes before serving.

## NUTRITION FACTS

Per Serving: 303 calories; 23.4 g fat; 1.1 g carbohydrates; 21.6 g protein; 144 mg cholesterol; 496 mg sodium.

## VEGETARIAN SANDWICH SPREAD

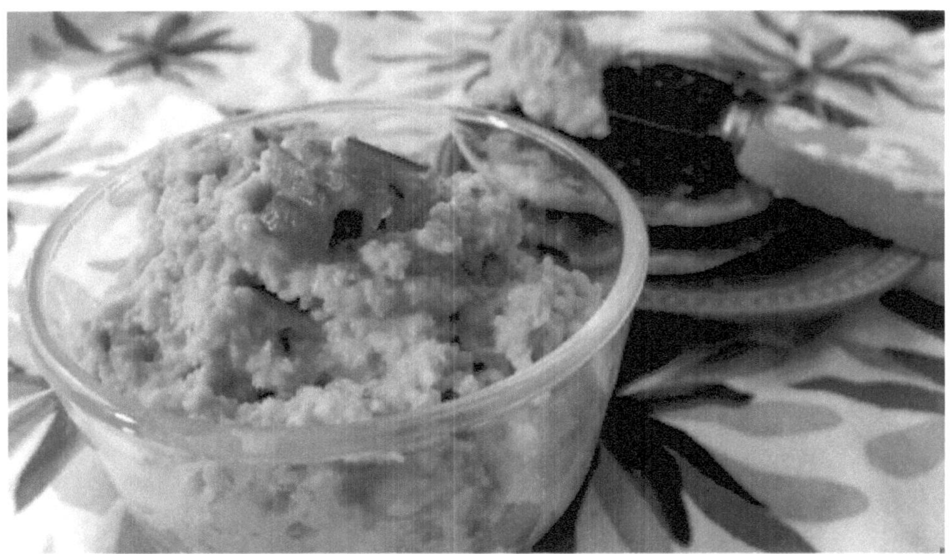

"Just like the meat spreads in the deli case. You can teach those veggie dogs new tricks!"

## INGREDIENTS

- 1 (19 ounce) can vegetarian hot dog links
- 3/4 cup sweet pickle relish
- 1 onion, chopped
- 1/2 cup mayonnaise

# DIRECTIONS

Prep
10 m

Ready In
10 m

Servings
12

- In a large bowl mash hot dog links using a potato masher or fork. Blend in relish, onion and mayonnaise.

## NUTRITION FACTS

Per Serving: 192 calories; 13.5 g fat; 7.8 g carbohydrates; 10.8 g protein; 3 mg cholesterol; 371 mg sodium.

# HEALTHIER BBQ PORK FOR SANDWICHES

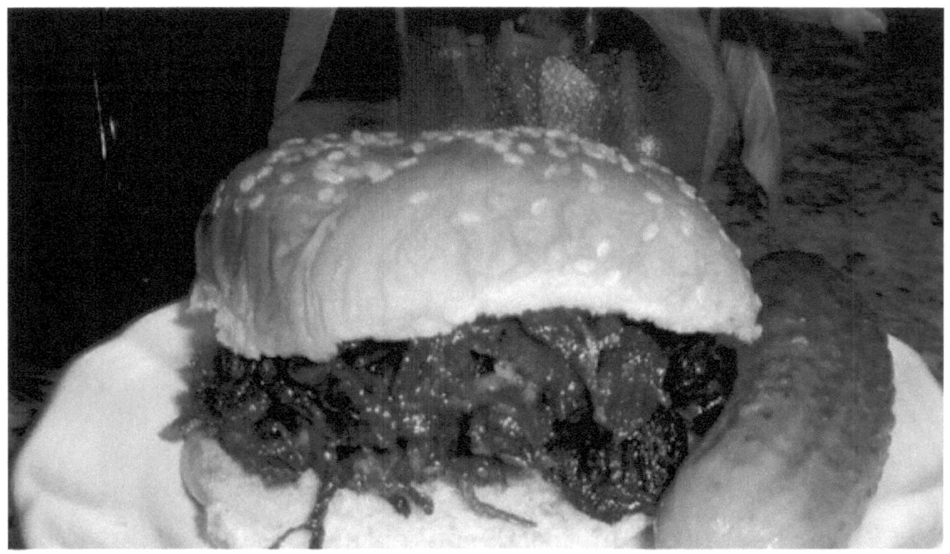

"This meat is so good for sandwiches. I like to add a little fiber to it with some carrots and cut out some sugar by using mesquite sauce."

## INGREDIENTS

- 1 (14 ounce) can beef broth
- 3 pounds boneless pork ribs
- 1 cup shredded carrot
- 4 1/2 fluid ounces barbeque sauce
- 4 1/2 ounces mesquite sauce

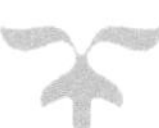

# DIRECTIONS

Prep
15 m

Cook
4 h 30 m

Ready In
4 h 45 m

Servings
12

- Pour beef broth into slow cooker and add pork ribs. Cook on High until meat shreds easily, about 4 hours. Remove meat and shred with two forks.
- Preheat oven to 350 degrees F (175 degrees C). Transfer shredded pork to a Dutch oven or skillet and stir in carrots, barbecue sauce, and mesquite sauce.
- Bake in preheated oven until heated through, about 30 minutes.

# NUTRITION FACTS

Per Serving: 322 calories; 18.1 g fat; 7.6 g carbohydrates; 30.3 g protein; 83 mg cholesterol; 541 mg sodium.

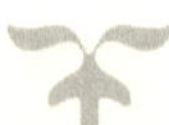

## VIRGINA'S TUNA SALAD

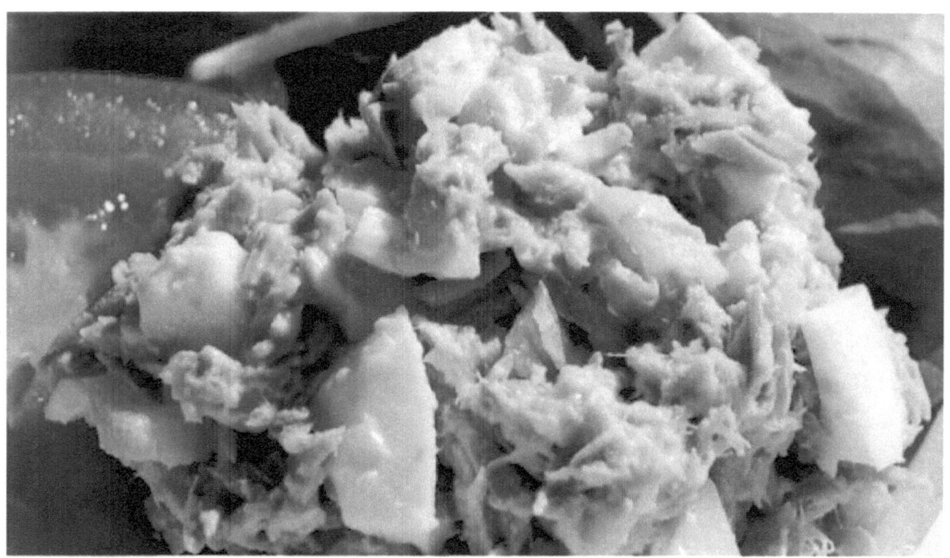

What can I eat for lunch instead of bread? Virginia's Tuna SaladThis was always You may also add grapes or chopped applies if you wish to eat for lunch.

# INGREDIENTS

- 1 egg
- 1 (5 ounce) can tuna, drained and flaked
- 3 tablespoons mayonnaise
- 2 stalks celery, chopped
- 2 tablespoons sweet pickle relish
- 1 pinch ground black pepper

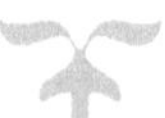

# DIRECTIONS

Prep
20 m

Cook
5 m

Ready In
40 m

Servings
4

- Place egg in a saucepan and cover with cold water. Bring water to a boil and immediately remove from heat. Cover and let egg stand in hot water for 10 to 12 minutes. Remove from hot water; cool for 5 minutes. Peel and chop into bite-sized pieces.
- In a medium bowl, mix together tuna and mayonnaise. Mix in egg, celery, relish, and black pepper.

# NUTRITION FACTS

Per Serving: 142 calories; 9.8 g fat; 3.9 g carbohydrates; 9.9 g protein; 60 mg cholesterol; 168 mg sodium.

# CHICKEN SALAD SPREAD

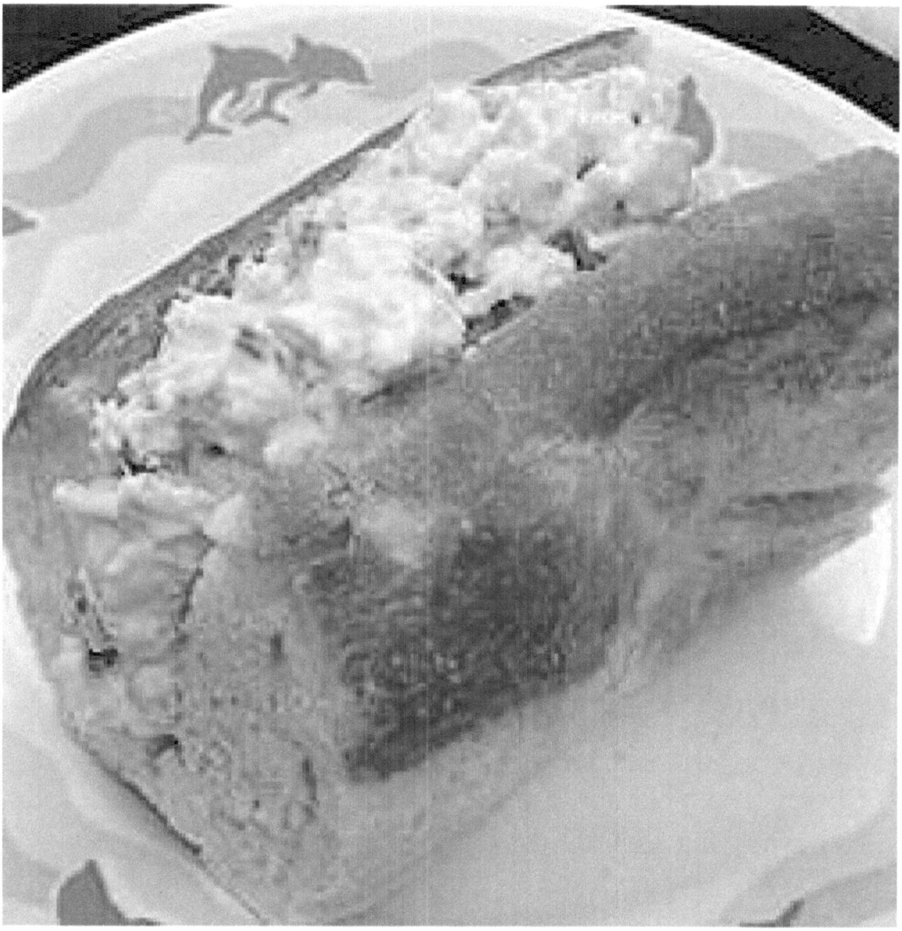

The chicken salad is quick and easy. If you want a little 'zip', add a few drops of hot sauce to the mixture! Serve on lettuce as a salad or on bread as a sandwich.

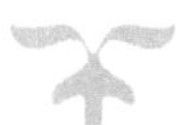

# INGREDIENTS

- 1 (10 ounce) can chicken chunks, drained
- ¼ cup chopped celery
- ⅓ cup low-fat mayonnaise
- ½ teaspoon onion powder
- ½ cup sweet pickles, chopped

# DIRECTIONS

Servings
4

- Combine the chicken meat, celery, mayonnaise, onion powder and sweet pickles.

# NUTRITION FACTS

Per Serving: 145 calories; 5.6 g total fat; 43 mg cholesterol; 476 mg sodium. 7.4 g carbohydrates; 15.3 g protein;

# SUSHI-INSPIRED TUNA SALAD

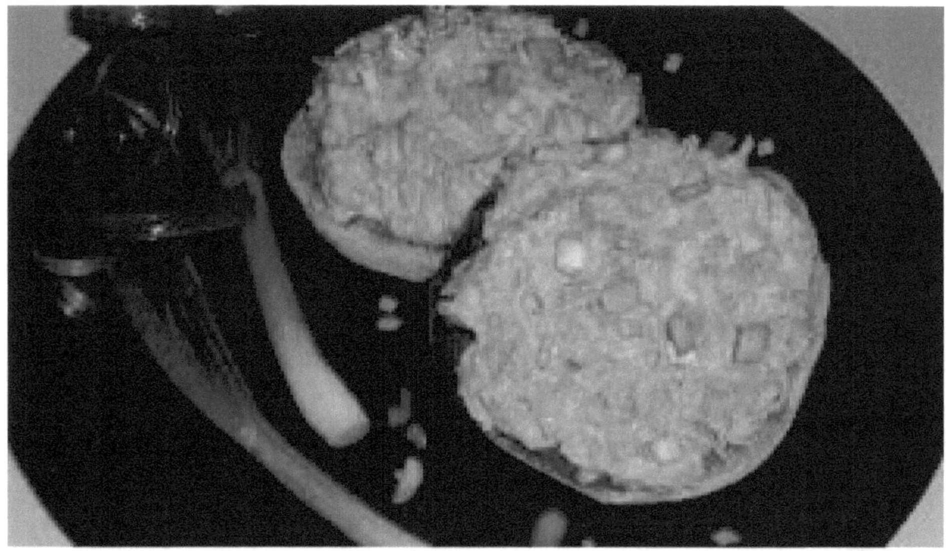

The clock strikes noon, and the hunger pangs have just started to gnaw at an empty stomach. There is the option of popping open a can of flakey dolphin-safe tuna and dumping it along with a heaping spoonful of thick mayonnaise into the bowl. A quick chop of pickle, half an onion, and maybe a celery stick on a cutting board is sure to give the inevitable mixture some texture and bit of briny flavor. Lastly, smear that creamy, crunchy, concoction on a slice of soft bread with a lettuce leaf and a slice of ripe tomato (just so it's well rounded) and top with another slice of bread.　Behold the classic tuna salad sandwich, a sandwich that has sated lunchtime hunger for decades. This is what comes to mind when I hear the term "tuna salad", but what I present to you is something completely different.

## INGREDIENTS

- 1 (5 ounce) can solid white tuna packed in water, drained
- 1/2 cup mayonnaise
- 1 tablespoon wasabi paste, or to taste
- 1 teaspoon minced fresh ginger root
- 1 tablespoon minced green onion

## DIRECTIONS

Prep
10 m

Ready In
10 m

Servings
2

- In a medium bowl, mix together the tuna, mayonnaise, wasabi paste, ginger and green onion. Serve on lettuce leaves or make a sandwich with white bread.

## NUTRITION FACTS

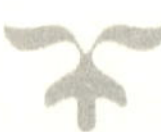

Per Serving: 492 calories; 44.2 g fat; 6.6 g carbohydrates; 16.6 g protein; 40 mg cholesterol; 502 mg sodium.

# SAVORY STUFFED CELERY BITES

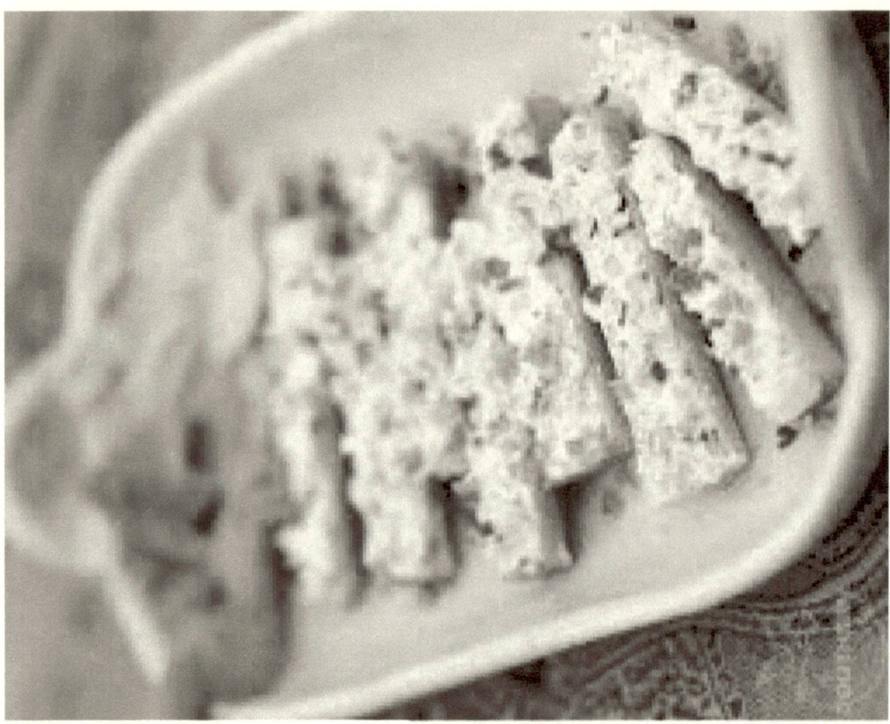

Anyone can make this simple, old-fashioned, and tasty appetizer of celery sticks stuffed with a cream cheese and green olive filling. The green celery and olives with red pimiento pieces look pretty on an appetizer tray, too.

# INGREDIENTS

- 1 bunch celery
- 1 (8 ounce) package cream cheese
- 1/4 cup chopped walnuts
- 20 small green olives
- 2 tablespoons sour cream

# DIRECTIONS

Servings
10

- Coarsely chop the olives. Separate and wash celery stalks. Cut stalks into bite sized pieces.
- Mix the cream cheese and sour cream together. Stir in the walnuts and chopped olives. Spread filling onto the celery pieces. It's also good on crackers.

# NUTRITION FACTS

Per Serving: 121 calories; 11.4 g fat; 2.8 g carbohydrates; 2.7 g protein; 26 mg cholesterol; 299 mg sodium.

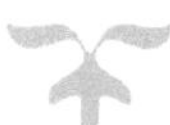

## BLACKBERRY SPINACH SALAD

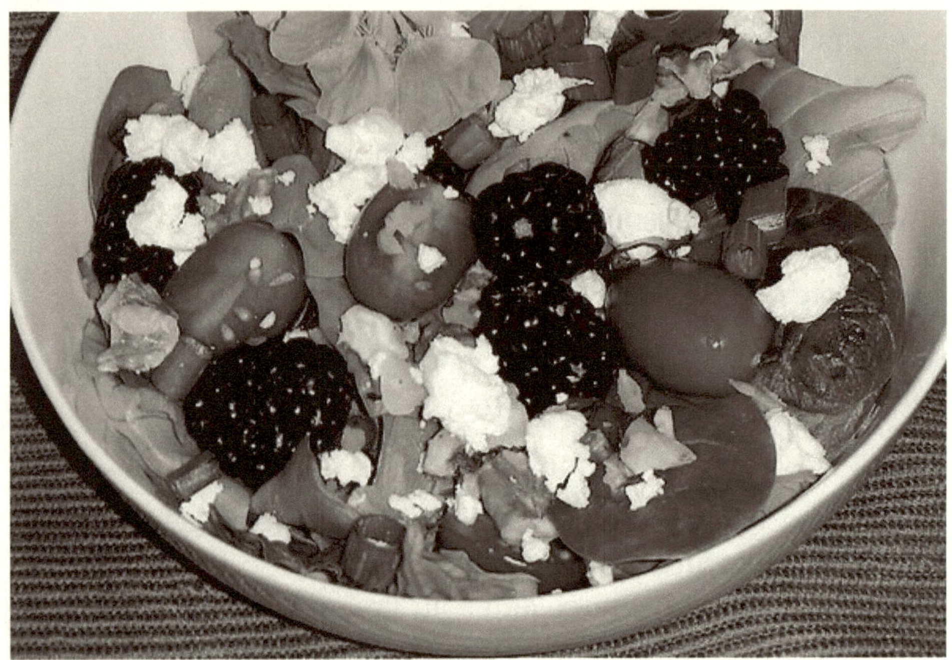

This is an excellent brunch salad that's very easy to throw together. This tastes great without a dressing, but some people like a bacon dressing or a nice balsamic vinegar.

## INGREDIENTS

- 3 cups baby spinach, rinsed and dried
- 1 pint fresh blackberries
- 6 ounces crumbled feta cheese
- 1 pint cherry tomatoes, halved

- 1 green onion, sliced
- ¼ cup finely chopped walnuts (optional)
- ½ cup edible flowers (optional)

## DIRECTIONS

Prep
10 m

Cook
5 m

Ready In
15 m

Servings
8

- In a large bowl, toss together baby spinach, blackberries, feta cheese, cherry tomatoes, green onion, and walnuts. Garnish with edible flowers.

## NUTRITION FACTS

Per Serving: 107 calories; 7.3 g total fat; 19 mg cholesterol; 250 mg sodium. 7.1 g carbohydrates; 4.8 g protein;

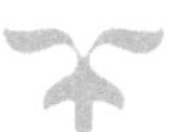

# FETA-STUFFED HAMBURGERS

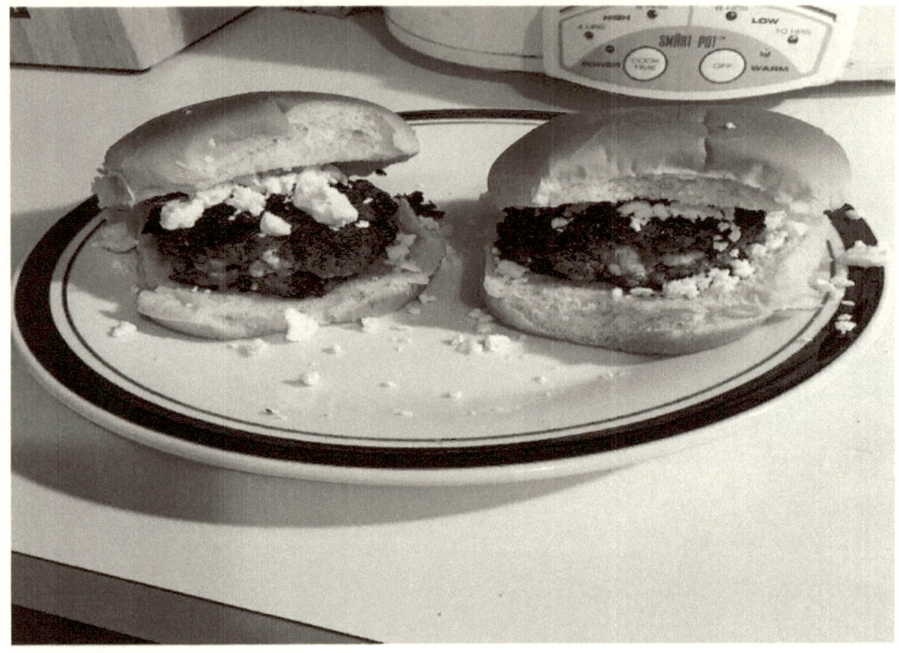

This is a great hamburger for the grill. Feta cheese gives it a rich and creamy taste.

## INGREDIENTS

- 1 pound lean ground beef
- ½ teaspoon Worcestershire sauce
- 1 teaspoon dried parsley
- salt and pepper to taste
- 1 cup crumbled feta cheese

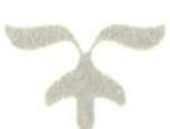

# DIRECTIONS

Prep
5 m

Cook
15 m

Ready In
20 m

Servings
4

- Preheat an outdoor grill for medium heat, and lightly oil the grate.

- Knead together the ground beef, Worcestershire sauce, parsley, salt, and pepper in a bowl. Form the mixture into 8 equal-sized balls; flatten to make thin patties. Place about 1/4 cup of feta cheese onto each of four of the patties. Top each of the patties with cheese with one of the patties without; press the edges together to seal the cheese into the center.

- Cook on the preheated grill until the burgers are cooked to your desired degree of doneness, 7 to 8 minutes per side for

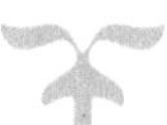

well done. An instant-read thermometer inserted into the center should read 160 degrees F (70 degrees C).

## NUTRITION FACTS

Per Serving: 386 calories; 27.2 g total fat; 135 mg cholesterol; 780 mg sodium. 2.8 g carbohydrates; 31 g protein;

# RED, WHITE AND BLUE BURGERS

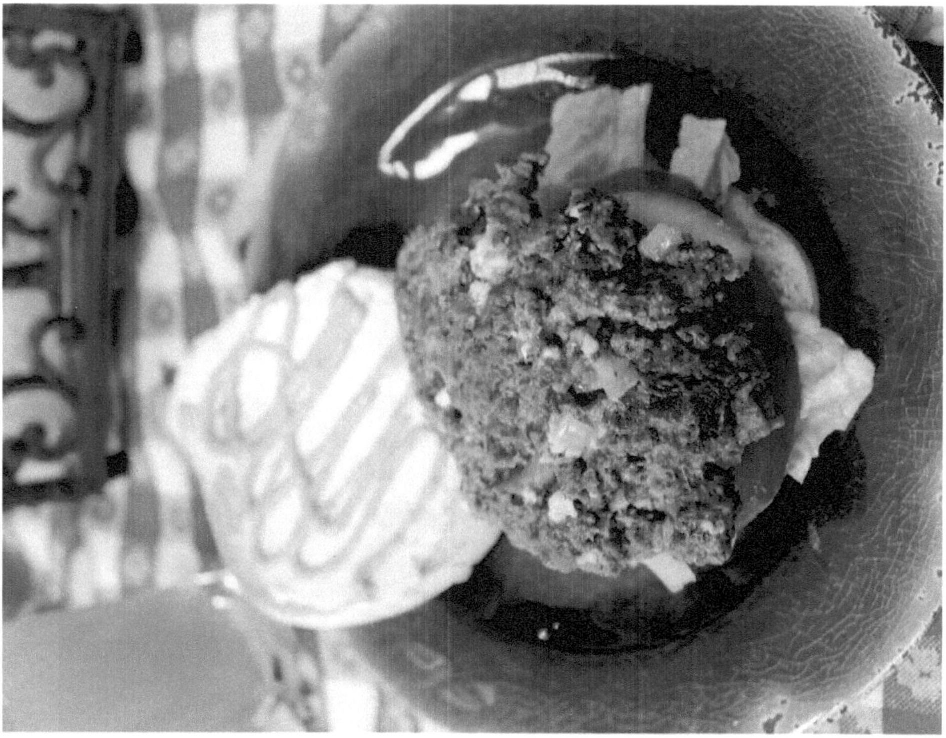

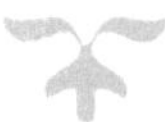

I get more requests to make this burger. They are to-die-for-juicy, and the flavor can't be beat. The onions cook on the inside of the burger. No need for toppings on these delicious burgers. I freeze extra single burgers in a sandwich bag for a quick week night meal. Enjoy the juiciness.

# INGREDIENTS

- 2 pounds ground beef sirloin
- 1 red onion, diced
- ½ (1 ounce) package dry ranch salad dressing mix
- 4 ounces crumbled blue cheese

# DIRECTIONS

Prep
5 m

Cook
20 m

Ready In
25 m

Servings
6

- Preheat an outdoor grill for medium-high heat, and lightly oil the grate.

- Lightly mix together the ground sirloin, onion, ranch salad dressing mix, and blue cheese in a bowl. Form into 6 patties.

- Grill the burgers for about 5 minutes per side on the prepared grill, until well done.

## NUTRITION FACTS

Per Serving: 372 calories; 23.9 g total fat; 120 mg cholesterol; 521 mg sodium. 3.3 g carbohydrates; 33.7 g protein;

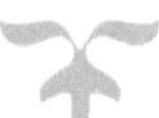

## CHICKEN WALNUT CHEESE WRAPPED IN BACON

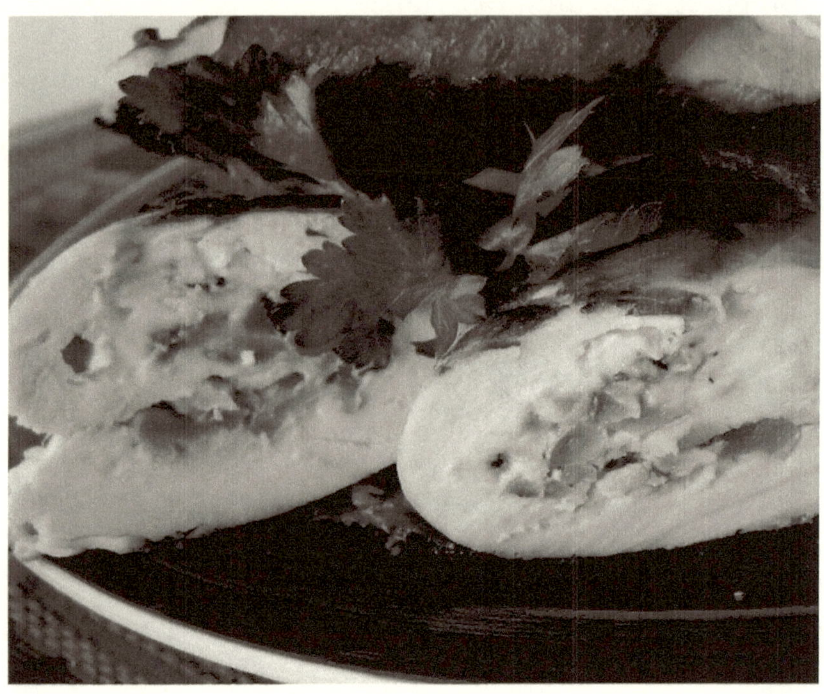

Devilishly good and (almost) paleo-approved! Use the leftover drippings to fry some side-dish veggies, or just drizzle on top of the completed chicken. Go ahead and modify the cheese; any stinky cheese will do. Can also substitute candied walnuts or pecans for standard walnuts for a unique sweet-and-savory flavor.

## INGREDIENTS

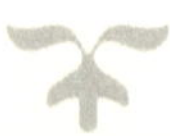

- 2 boneless, skinless chicken breasts, halved horizontally
- 8 ounces crumbled blue cheese
- 6 ounces walnut halves
- 8 slices bacon

## DIRECTIONS

Prep
20 m

Cook
35 m

Ready In
55 m

Servings
4

- Preheat oven to 350 degrees F (175 degrees C).

- Pound chicken slices until they are even in thickness and about 1/4-inch thick. Spread blue cheese and walnuts on top of each chicken piece. Roll chicken breasts over filling.

- Place 2 bacon slices side by side on a work surface. Place each chicken roll at one end of bacon slices and roll bacon around chicken; secure with toothpicks. Repeat with remaining chicken rolls and bacon.

- Heat a skillet to medium-high heat and cook bacon-wrapped chicken rolls in the hot skillet until the bacon is browned and crisp, 4 to 5 minutes per side. Transfer chicken rolls to preheated oven; bake until chicken is no longer pink in the center and the juices run clear, 25 to 35 minutes.

## NUTRITION FACTS

Per Serving: 637 calories; 52.8 g total fat; 93 mg cholesterol; 1238 mg sodium. 7.4 g carbohydrates; 36.8 g protein;

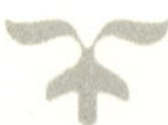

# PEACHY CHICKEN SALAD

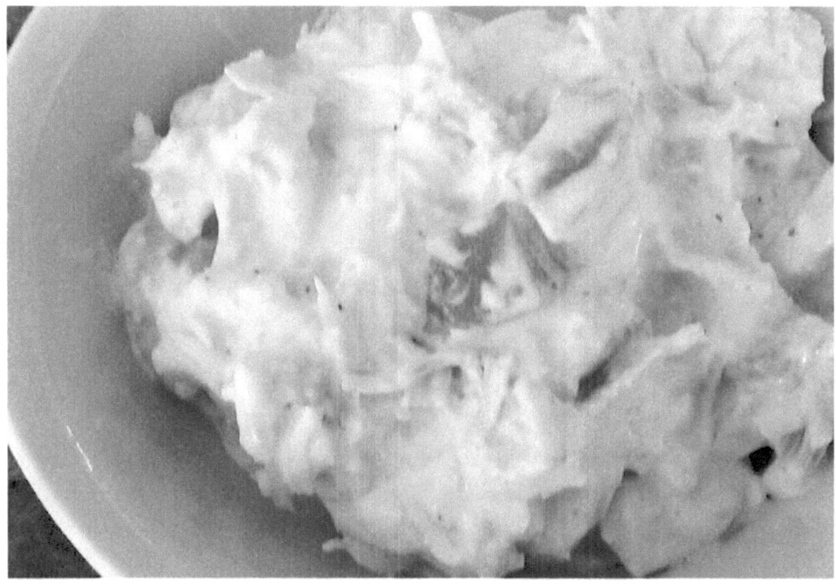

Fresh and fruity, this creamy, peach dotted chicken salad marries sweet and savory to a palette-pleasing effect.

## INGREDIENTS

- 1 cup mayonnaise
- ¼ cup peach juice
- ⅔ cup whipped heavy cream
- salt and pepper to taste
- 4 cups cubed, cooked chicken
- 3 cups pitted and diced fresh peaches

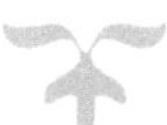

# DIRECTIONS

Prep
20 m

Ready In
20 m

Servings
6

- In a large bowl, whisk together the mayonnaise, peach juice and whipped cream. Add salt and pepper to taste. Stir in chicken and peaches and chill until ready to serve.

# NUTRITION FACTS

Per Serving: 535 calories; 45.7 g total fat; 105 mg cholesterol; 279 mg sodium. 6.9 g carbohydrates; 23.7 g protein;

# CHIPOTLE BLUE CHEESE DIP

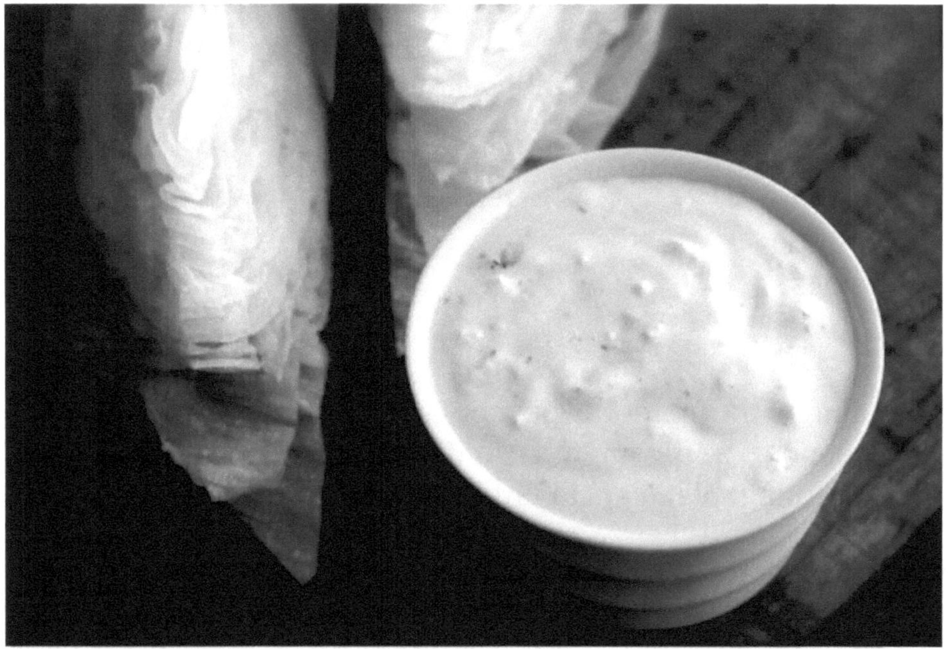

This spicy dip for tortilla chips is also a great sauce for grilled chicken or hamburgers.

## INGREDIENTS

- 1 (7 ounce) can chipotle peppers in adobo sauce
- 1 cup mayonnaise
- 2 tablespoons milk
- 1 ½ cups chunky blue cheese dressing

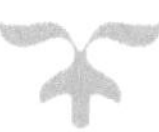

# DIRECTIONS

Prep
10 m

Ready In
10 m

Servings
10

- Puree the chipotle peppers with the adobo sauce in a blender until smooth. Add the mayonnaise, milk, and dressing; blend again until thoroughly mixed.

## NUTRITION FACTS

Per Serving: 354 calories; 37.1 g total fat; 15 mg cholesterol; 617 mg sodium. 4.8 g carbohydrates; 2.1 g protein;

# SPINACH SALAD WITH EASE

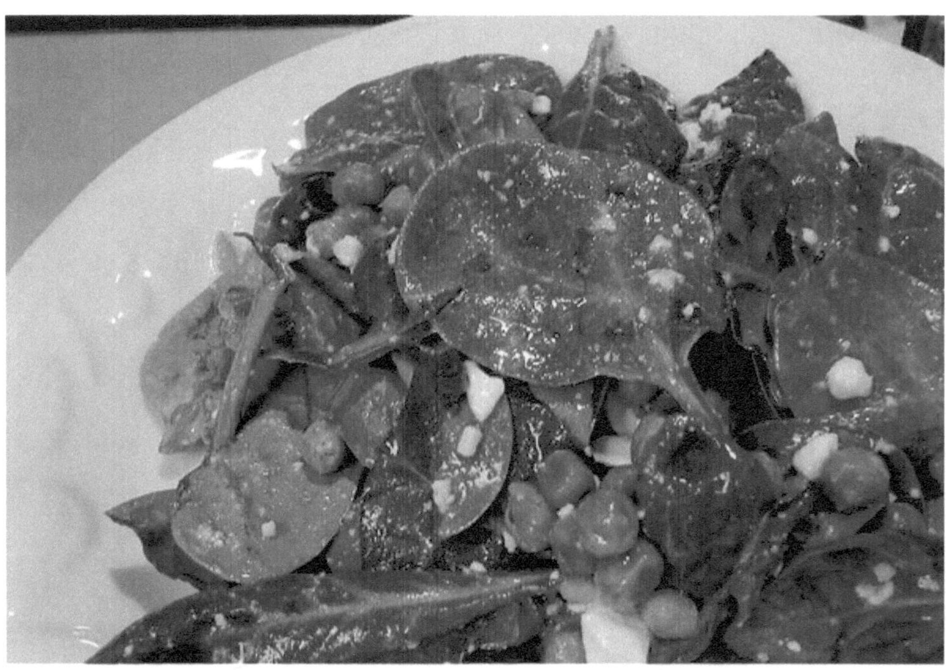

A simple, fresh salad. It comes together in less than 5 minutes. The perfect complement to almost any robust dish.

## INGREDIENTS

- 1 (10 ounce) package pre-washed fresh spinach
- 1 cup fresh green peas
- ¼ cup olive oil

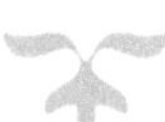

- 1 ½ lemons, juiced
- ¼ cup crumbled feta cheese
- salt and pepper to taste

# DIRECTIONS

Prep
5 m

Cook
0 m

Ready In
5 m

Servings
8

- In a large bowl, toss together the spinach, peas and olive oil until evenly coated. Add the lemon juice, feta and salt and pepper, and toss again.

# NUTRITION FACTS

Per Serving: 198 calories; 16 g total fat; 8 mg cholesterol; 163 mg sodium. 12.5 g carbohydrates; 5.8 g protein;

## CURRY CHICKEN SALAD

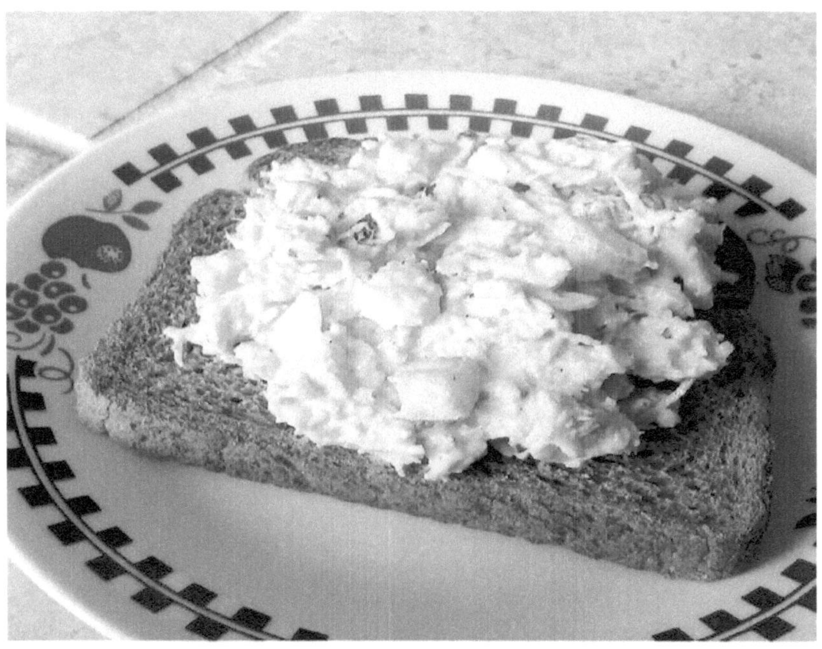

A cold chicken salad spread ideal for a sandwich. Serve on bread with lettuce, and enjoy!

# INGREDIENTS

- 3 cooked skinless, boneless chicken breast halves, chopped
- 3 stalks celery, chopped
- ½ cup low-fat mayonnaise
- 2 teaspoons curry powder

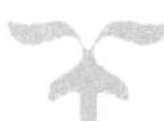

## DIRECTIONS

Prep
10 m

Cook
0 m

Ready In
10 m

Servings
6

- In a medium bowl, stir together the chicken, celery, mayonnaise, and curry powder.

## NUTRITION FACTS

Per Serving: 77 calories; 1.6 g total fat; 37 mg cholesterol; 46 mg sodium. 1 g carbohydrates; 14 g protein;

# LOOSEMEAT SANDWICHES II

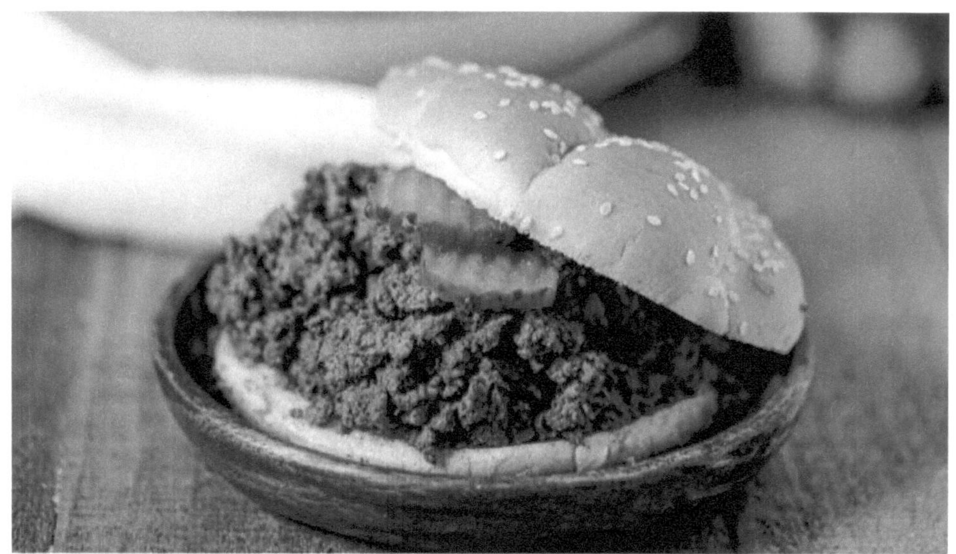

Loose Meat Sandwiches are flavorful Midwestern chopped meat burgers made with seasoned beef, Worcestershire sauce and onion, topped with dill pickles.

## INGREDIENTS

- 1 pound lean ground beef
- 1 (10.75 ounce) can condensed chicken gumbo soup

## DIRECTIONS

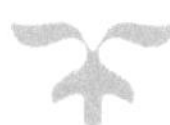

Prep
15 m

Cook
0 m

Ready In
15 m

Servings
6

- In large skillet over medium heat, cook ground beef until brown, 5 to 10 minutes. Drain. Return meat to skillet, with soup. Simmer until heated through, 5 minutes. Serve hot.

## NUTRITION FACTS

Per Serving:167 calories; 9.8 g total fat; 51 mg cholesterol; 432 mg sodium. 3.4 g carbohydrates; 15.5 g protein;

# BOLOGNA SALAD SANDWICH SPREAD

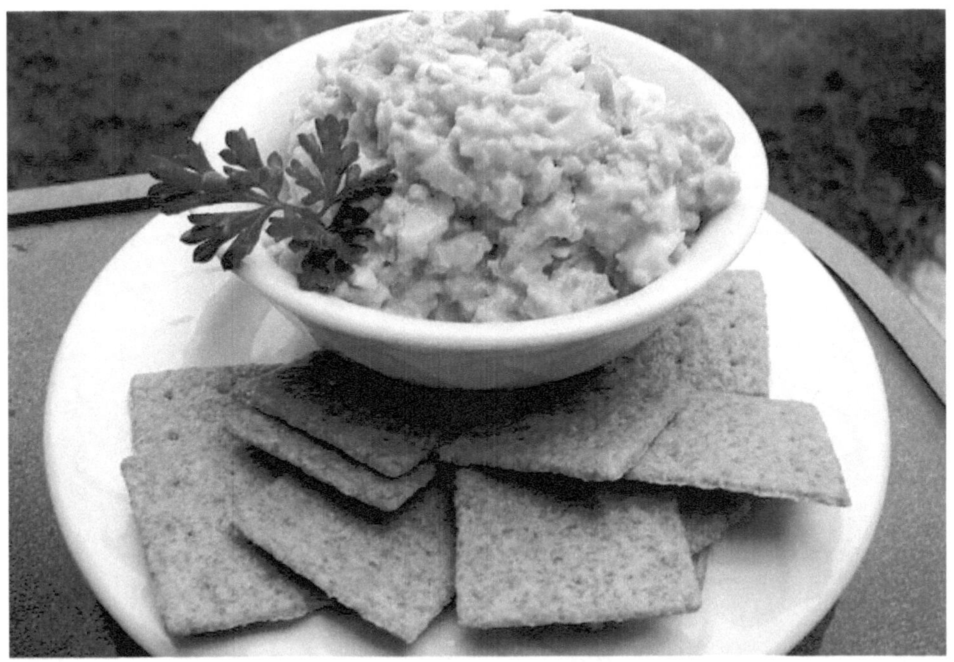

Sweet relish and eggs round out the flavor of bologna in this simple but delicious spread. Serve it on cocktail toast, or use it in sandwiches. The amount of egg, creamy salad dressing and relish should be adjusted to taste.

## INGREDIENTS

- 4 eggs
- 1 (16 ounce) package bologna

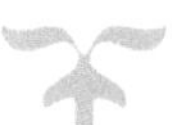

- 1 (16 ounce) jar creamy salad dressing
- 1 cup sweet pickle relish

## DIRECTIONS

Prep
20 m

Cook
2 hr 20 m

Ready In
2 hr 40 m

Servings
48

- Place eggs in a medium saucepan and cover with cold water. Bring water to a boil and immediately remove from heat. Cover and let eggs stand in hot water for 10 to 12 minutes. Remove from hot water, cool, peel and chop.

- Grind the bologna and eggs in a meat grinder with a medium blade.

- In a large bowl, mix the bologna mixture with desired amount of creamy salad dressing and desired amount of sweet pickle relish. Refrigerate 2 to 3 hours, or until chilled.

# NUTRITION FACTS

Per Serving:64 calories; 4.8 g total fat; 24 mg cholesterol; 236 mg sodium. 3.1 g carbohydrates; 2 g protein;

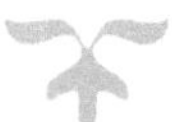

# PESTO TUNA SALAD WITH SUN-DRIED TOMATOES

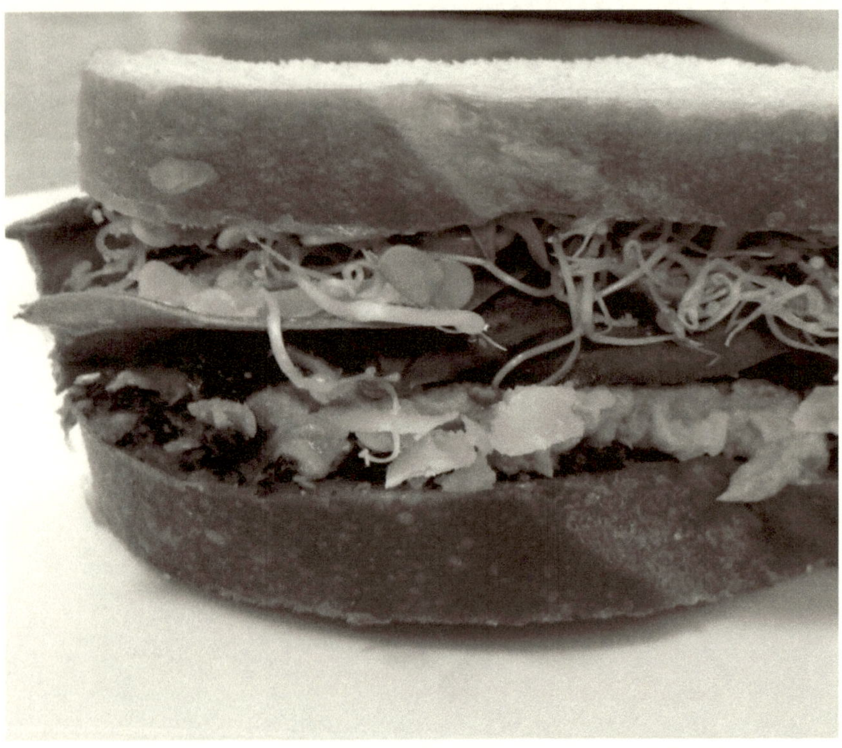

Sun Dried Tomatoes and Basil Pesto Tuna Salad – Combined with delicious basil pesto and flavorful sun dried tomatoes, this tuna salad is about to become your next favorite salad recipe that is perfect for any summer barbeque or just for lunch!

# INGREDIENTS

- 1 (5 ounce) can canned tuna
- ¼ cup prepared basil pesto sauce
- 6 oil-packed sun-dried tomatoes, drained and diced
- 2 tablespoons mayonnaise
- 2 tablespoons grated Parmesan cheese

# DIRECTIONS

Prep
15 m

Cook
0 m

Ready In
15 m

Servings
2

- In a bowl, mix the tuna, pesto, sun-dried tomatoes, mayonnaise, and Parmesan cheese. Cover, and refrigerate until ready to serve.

# NUTRITION FACTS

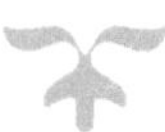

Per Serving:368 calories; 28.4 g total fat; 39 mg cholesterol; 448 mg sodium. 4.8 g carbohydrates; 24.2 g protein;

# CRAB LEGS WITH GARLIC BUTTER SAUCE

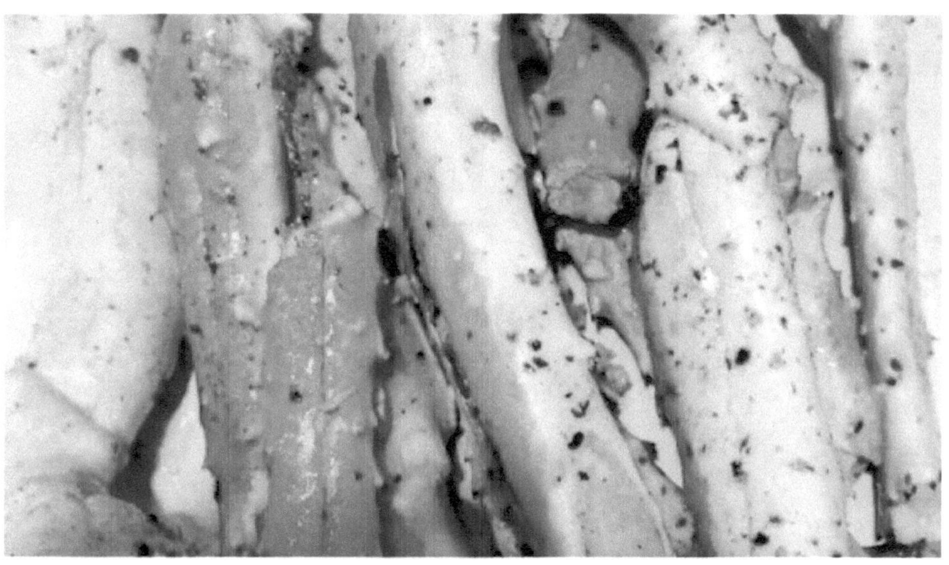

These crab legs are steamed to perfection, then tossed in a flavorful garlic butter sauce. A simple, yet satisfying way to enjoy fresh seafood, and it takes just minutes to put together! Crab legs make for a great appetizer or main course option.

## INGREDIENTS

- 1 pound Snow Crab clusters, thawed if necessary
- 1/4 cup butter
- 1 clove garlic, minced

- 1 1/2 teaspoons dried parsley
- 1/8 teaspoon salt
- 1/4 teaspoon fresh-ground black pepper

## DIRECTIONS

Prep
5 m

Cook
15 m

Ready In
20 m

Servings
2

- Cut a slit, length-wise, into the shell of each piece of crab.
- Melt the butter in a large skillet over medium heat; cook the garlic in the butter until translucent; stir in the parsley, salt, and pepper. Continue to heat mixture until bubbling. Add the crab legs; toss to coat; allow to simmer in the butter mixture until completely heated, 5 to 6 minutes.

## NUTRITION FACTS

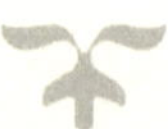

Per Serving: 520 calories; 37.5 g fat; 1 g carbohydrates; 43.6 g protein; 274 mg cholesterol; 1031 mg sodium.

# BEER BRATS

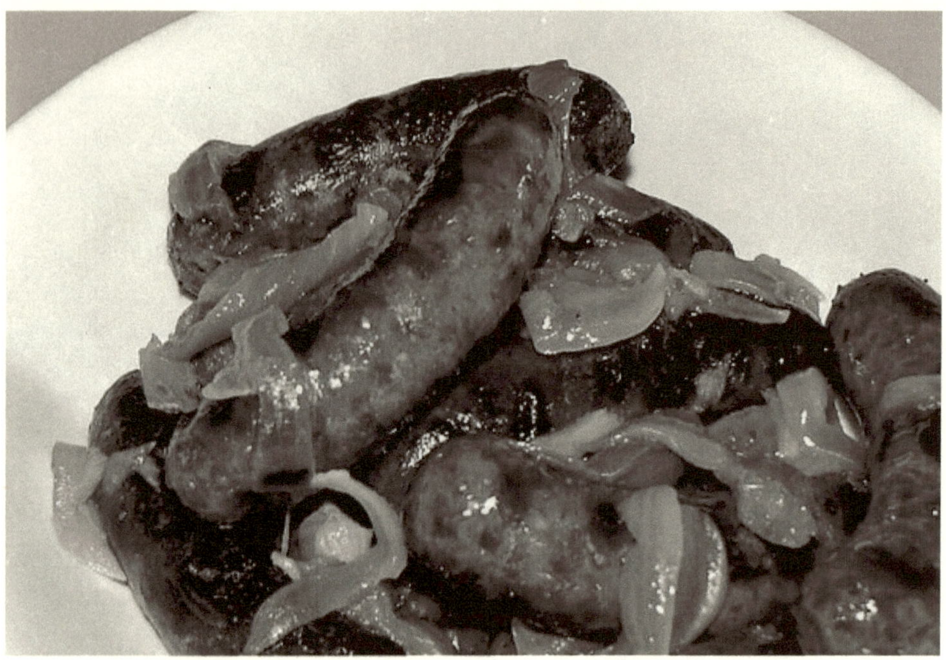

These awesome beer brats are boiled and then put on the grill!

## INGREDIENTS

- 4 (12 ounce) cans beer
- 1 large onion, diced
- 10 bratwurst
- 2 teaspoons red pepper flakes
- 1 teaspoon garlic powder

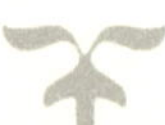

- 1 teaspoon salt and ½ teaspoon ground black pepper

## DIRECTIONS

Prep
5 m

Cook
20 m

Ready In
25 m

Servings
10

- Preheat an outdoor grill for medium-high heat. When hot, lightly oil grate.

- Combine the beer and onions in a large pot; bring to a boil. Submerge the bratwurst in the beer; add the red pepper flakes, garlic powder, salt, and pepper. Reduce heat to medium and cook another 10 to 12 minutes. Remove the bratwurst from the beer mixture; reduce heat to low, and continue cooking the onions.

- Cook the bratwurst on the preheated grill, turning once, 5 to 10 minutes. Serve with the beer mixture as a topping or side.

## NUTRITION FACTS

Per Serving: 382 calories; 27.4 g total fat; 69 mg cholesterol; 1031 mg sodium. 9.7 g carbohydrates; 13.8 g protein;

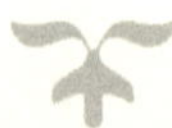

## SLOW COOKER MACHACA

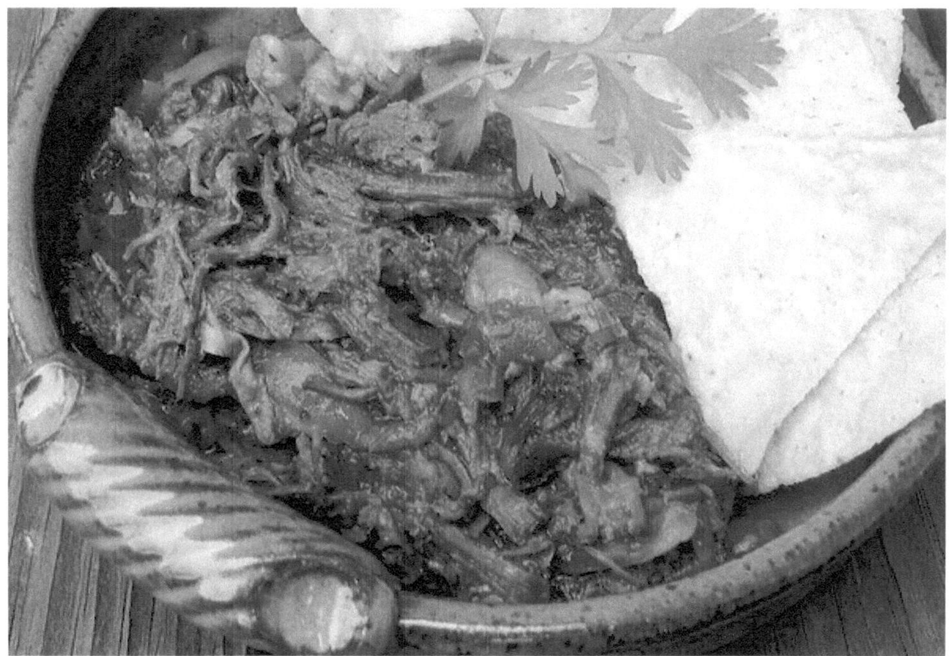

Beef and pork cooked in a slow cooker overnight creates the most tender Mexican meat filling you'll ever have. Serve with tortillas, cheese, and sour cream.

## INGREDIENTS

- 3 pounds beef rump roast
- 3 pounds pork loin roast
- 2 teaspoons salt
- 1 teaspoon ground black pepper

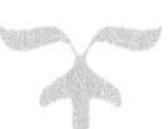

- 2 (14.5 ounce) cans green enchilada sauce
- 2 (4 ounce) cans diced green chiles

# DIRECTIONS

Prep
5 m

Cook
12 hr

Ready In
12 hr 5 m

Servings
10

- Season beef roast and pork loin with the salt and pepper. Place seasoned beef and pork in a slow cooker.

- Set slow cooker to Low. Cover, and cook overnight or 8 to 10 hours. Drain the juices and shred the meat into strands. Return the meat to the slow cooker; pour the enchilada sauce and green chiles in with the shredded meat and cook on Low another 4 to 8 hours.

# NUTRITION FACTS

Per Serving: 563 calories; 32.5 g total fat; 170 mg cholesterol; 1074 mg sodium. 6.9 g carbohydrates; 57.3 g protein;

# PINWHEELS

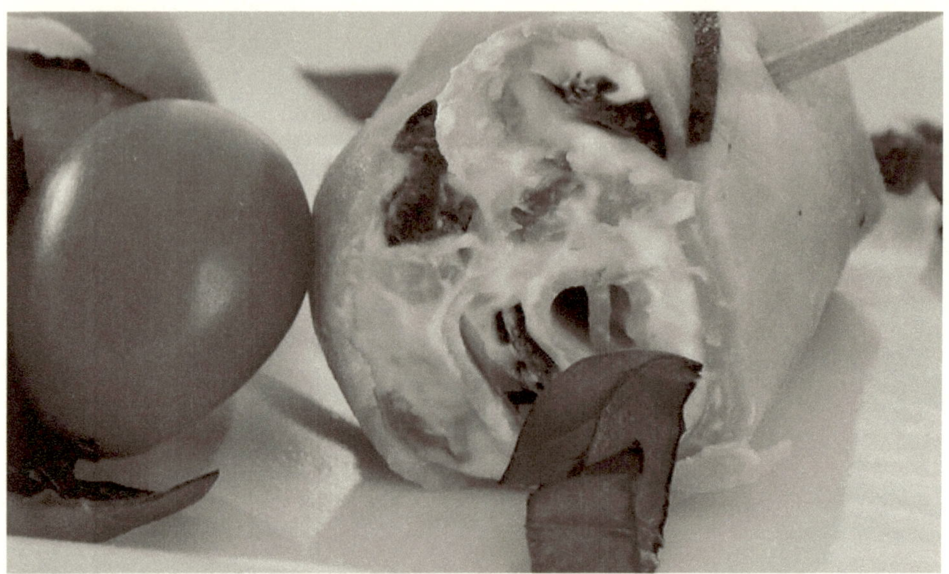

Flavored cream cheese spread on lunch meat of choice, rolled up, and sliced into pinwheels secured with toothpicks.

## INGREDIENTS

- 1 (8 ounce) package cream cheese, softened
- 1 tablespoon prepared horseradish
- 1 tablespoon Worcestershire sauce
- 2 tablespoons chopped sweet pickles
- 1 (2.25 ounce) can black olives, drained and chopped

## DIRECTIONS

Prep
10 m

Cook
0 m

Ready In
10 m

Servings
12

- In a medium bowl, mix together cream cheese, horseradish, Worcestershire sauce, sweet pickles and black olives. Chill in the refrigerator until ready to use.

## NUTRITION FACTS

Per Serving: 75 calories; 7.1 g total fat; 21 mg cholesterol; 129 mg sodium. 1.8 g carbohydrates; 1.5 g protein;

## PICKLE ROLLUPS

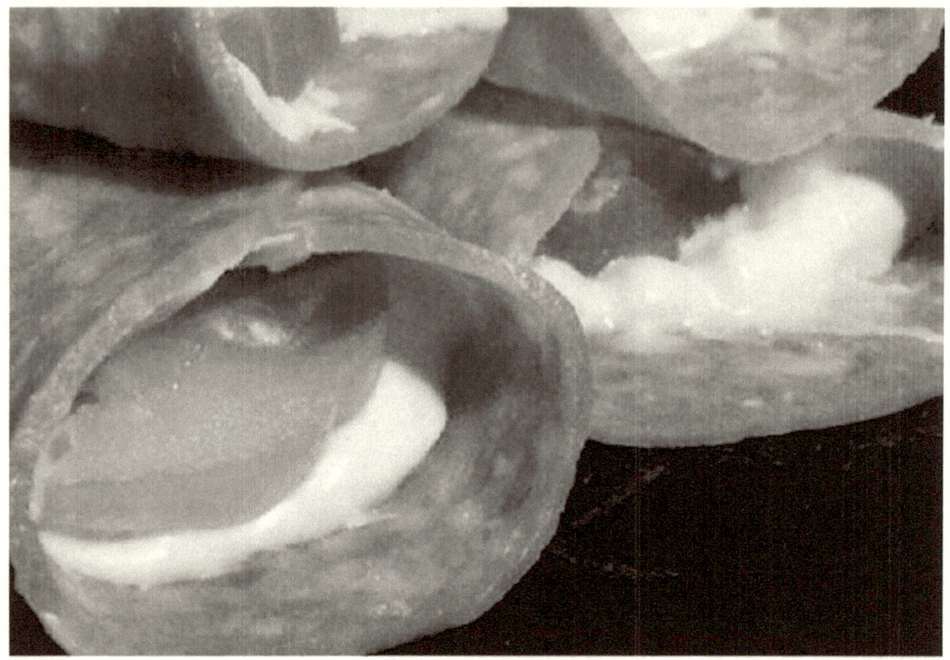

A quick finger food that everybody loves, and you can vary the meat according to your taste. My friends like salami or corned beef best.

## INGREDIENTS

- 16 ounces sliced pastrami
- 2 (8 ounce) packages cream cheese, softened
- 1 (16 ounce) jar dill pickles, cut into strips lengthwise

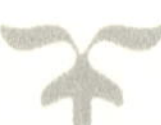

# DIRECTIONS

Prep
10 m

Cook
0 m

Ready In
10 m

Servings
10

- Spread cream cheese over a meat slice to cover. Place a pickle piece on one end, and roll the meat up. Repeat with remaining ingredients. Cut into 1 1/2 inch pieces, and chill until ready to serve.

# NUTRITION FACTS

Per Serving: 230 calories; 18.3 g total fat; 80 mg cholesterol; 1103 mg sodium. 3.2 g carbohydrates; 13.4 g protein;

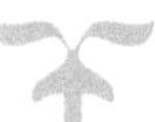

## HUMMUS

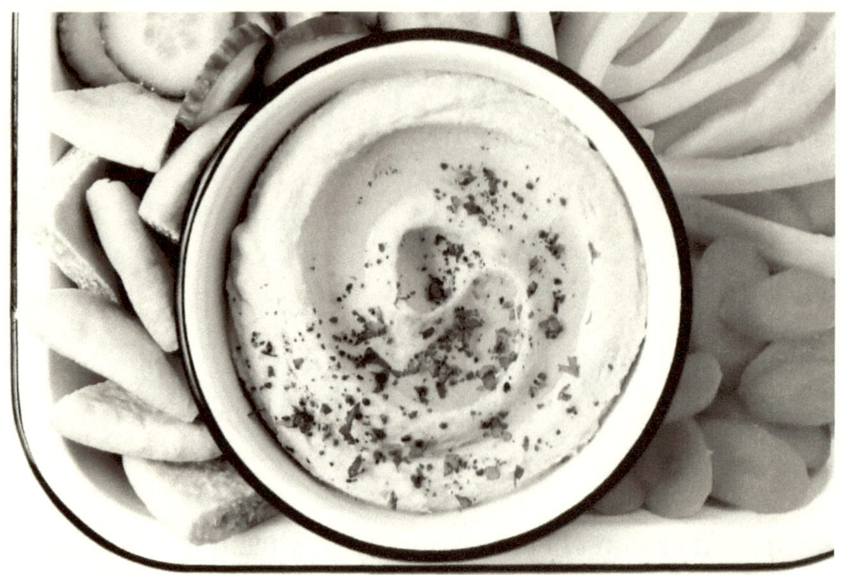

A straightforward hummus that may be augmented with roasted red peppers or olives. Serve with crackers, flat breads or on a pita with sprouts for a great light lunch.

## INGREDIENTS

- 2 (15.5 ounce) cans garbanzo beans, drained
- 4 tablespoons lemon juice
- 6 cloves garlic, peeled and crushed
- 3 tablespoons tahini
- ¼ teaspoon crushed red pepper

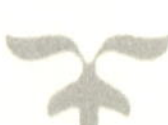

# DIRECTIONS

Prep
20 m

Cook
 0 m

Ready In
20 m

Servings
16

- Place garbanzo beans in a food processor and blend into a spreadable paste. Mix in lemon juice, garlic, tahini and crushed red pepper. Blend until smooth, using more lemon juice if consistency is too thick.

# NUTRITION FACTS

Per Serving: 34 calories; 0.9 g total fat; 0 mg cholesterol; 67 mg sodium. 5.5 g carbohydrates; 1.3 g protein;

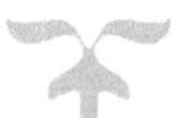

# VEGETABLE BEEF SOUP WITH GROUND BEEF

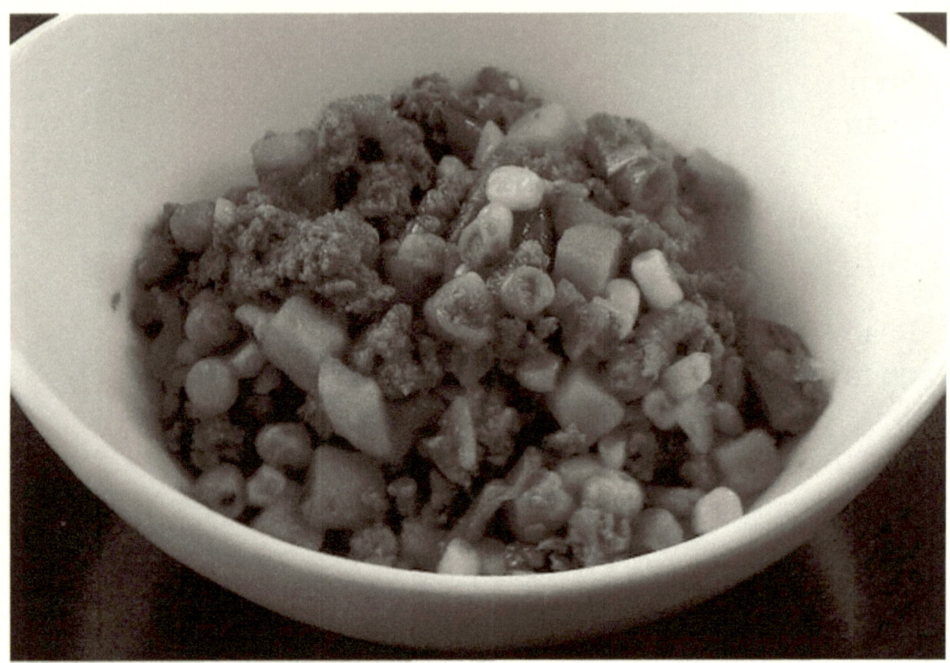

Simple! Brown the meat, and throw it all together into one pot. Serve soup with a cake of corn bread or grilled cheese sandwiches on a cold winter night. You will feel warm all over.

## INGREDIENTS

- 2 pounds lean ground beef
- 4 (15 ounce) cans mixed vegetables
- 4 (16 ounce) cans diced tomatoes
- 1 onion, chopped

- ground black pepper to taste
- salt to taste

# DIRECTIONS

Prep
20 m

Cook
3 hr

Ready In
3 hr 20 m

Servings
16

- In a large soup pot, cook ground meat over medium heat until browned. Drain grease from the pot.

- Add chopped onion, mixed vegetables, and tomatoes. Give it a stir. Reduce heat, and simmer for about 3 to 4 hours. Season to taste with salt and pepper.

## NUTRITION FACTS

Per Serving: 213 calories; 12 g total fat; 43 mg cholesterol; 537 mg sodium. 11.7 g carbohydrates; 12.5 g protein;

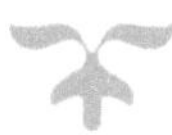

# BROILED SALMON PESTO

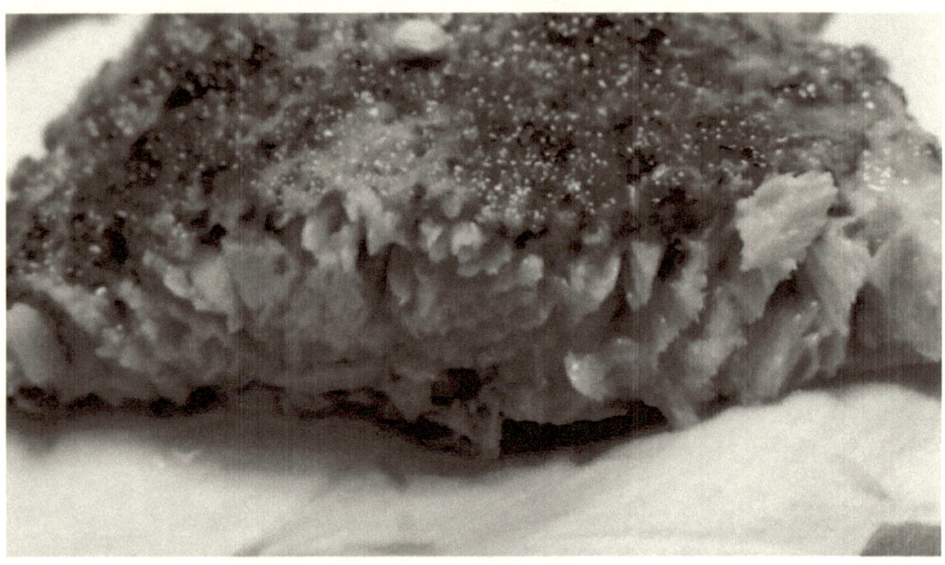

"This salmon is coated with a thick layer of pesto, sort of like icing on a cake. The prepared side is then placed under the broiler, and the pesto forms a browned crust. Equally good cold--the entire dish can be made a day in advance for cold service, or the leftovers served cold at lunch the next day. Goes well with rosemary and garlic roasted red potatoes and any green vegetable."

## INGREDIENTS

- 2 pounds salmon fillets
- 2 lemons

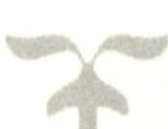

- 1 1/2 cups pesto
- 1/2 cup white wine

## DIRECTIONS

Prep
10 m

Cook
15 m

Ready In
40 m

Servings
4

- Lightly oil a baking pan large enough to accommodate the fish. Place salmon in pan skin side down. Run finger over flesh to make sure all bones have been removed. Use pliers to pull out any that remain. Squeeze juice of one lemon and white wine over fish. Marinate 15 minutes.
- Preheat broiler.
- Coat the top side of the fish with thick layer of pesto. It should be between an 1/8th to a 1/4 of an inch thick, and cover the surface of the fish.
- Place fish under the broiler about nine inches from heat source. Broil for 8 to 10 minutes per inch of thickness, or

until fish flakes and flesh is opaque. Pesto should have formed a heavily browned crust. Remove from the oven, and set aside for a few minutes. Squeeze half of second lemon over fish. Slice remaining lemon half into thin slices. Place lemon slices on individual servings, or arrange on the whole flank if serving at the table.

## NUTRITION FACTS

Per Serving: 917 calories; 67.4 g fat; 12.7 g carbohydrates; 62.6 g protein; 164 mg cholesterol; 851 mg sodium.

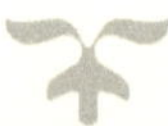

# DINNER

# SLOW COOKER POT ROAST

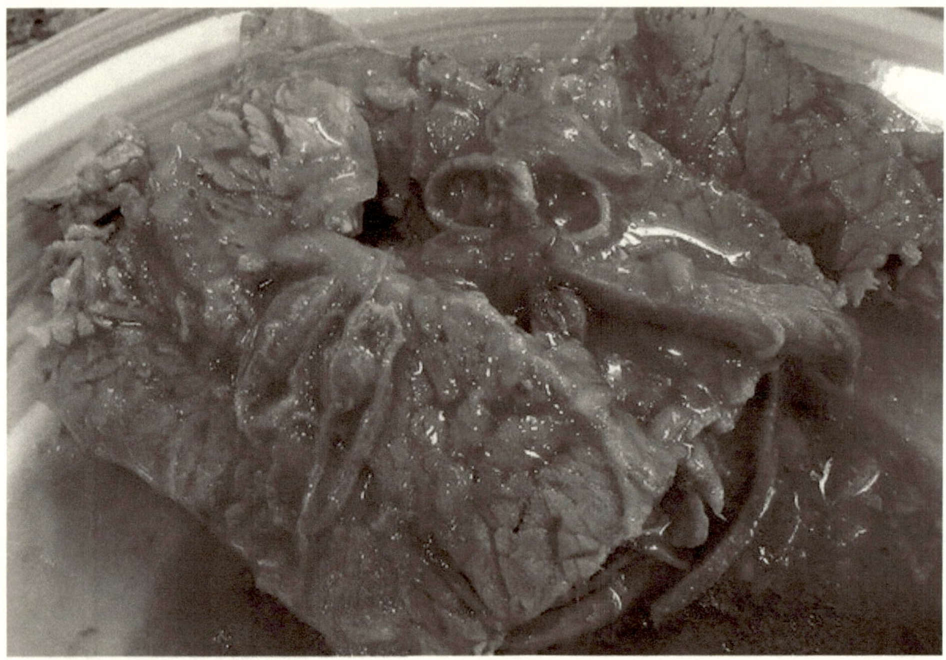

This is a very easy recipe for a delicious pot roast. It makes its own gravy. It's designed especially for the working person who does not have time to cook all day, but it tastes like you did. You'll want the cut to be between 5 and 6 pounds.

## INGREDIENTS

- 2 (10.75 ounce) cans condensed cream of mushroom soup
- 1 (1 ounce) package dry onion soup mix

- 1 ¼ cups water
- 5 ½ pounds pot roast

# DIRECTIONS

Prep
10 m

Cook
8 hr

Ready In
8 hr 10 m

Servings
12

- In a slow cooker, mix cream of mushroom soup, dry onion soup mix and water. Place pot roast in slow cooker and coat with soup mixture.

- Cook on High setting for 3 to 4 hours, or on Low setting for 8 to 9 hours.

# NUTRITION FACTS

Per Serving: 426 calories; 23.7 g total fat; 127 mg cholesterol; 639 mg sodium. 4.9 g carbohydrates; 45.6 g protein;

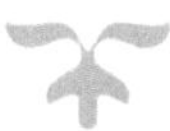

# GARLIC CHICKEN

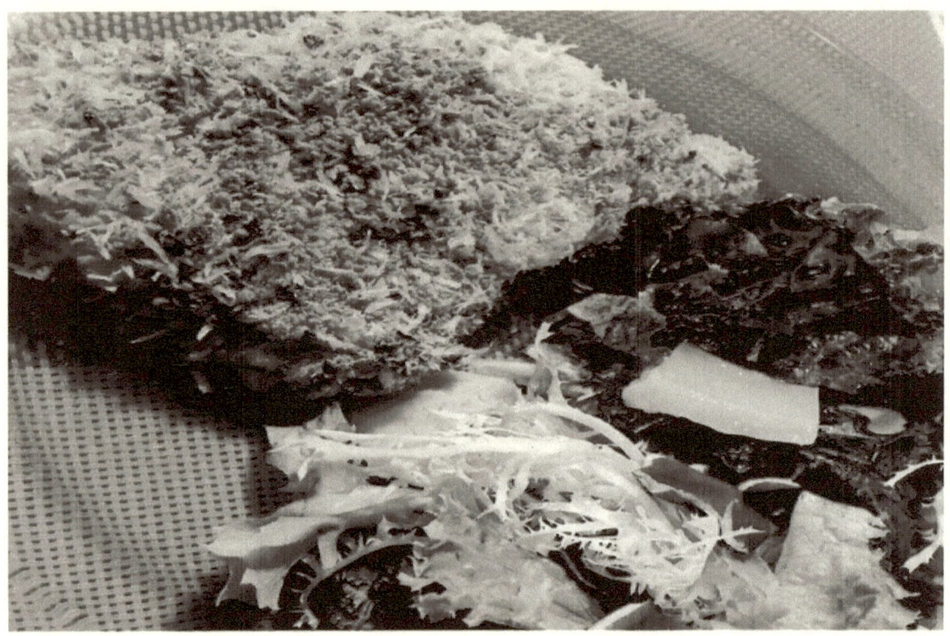

Simple to make, just dip and bake! Garlicky goodness in a breaded chicken dish. Yum!

## INGREDIENTS

- ¼ cup olive oil
- 2 cloves garlic, crushed
- ¼ cup Italian-seasoned bread crumbs
- ¼ cup grated Parmesan cheese
- 4 skinless, boneless chicken breast halves

## DIRECTIONS

Prep
20 m

Cook
35 m

Ready In
55 m

Servings
4

- Preheat oven to 425 degrees F (220 degrees C).

- Heat olive oil and garlic in a small saucepan over low heat until warmed, 1 to 2 minutes. Transfer garlic and oil to a shallow bowl.

- Combine bread crumbs and Parmesan cheese in a separate shallow bowl.

- Dip chicken breasts in the olive oil-garlic mixture using tongs; transfer to bread crumb mixture and turn to evenly coat. Transfer coated chicken to a shallow baking dish.

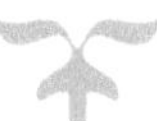

- Bake in the preheated oven until no longer pink and juices run clear, 30 to 35 minutes. An instant-read thermometer inserted into the center should read at least 165 degrees F (74 degrees C).

## NUTRITION FACTS

Per Serving: 300 calories; 16.8 g total fat; 73 mg cholesterol; 261 mg sodium. 5.7 g carbohydrates; 30.3 g protein;

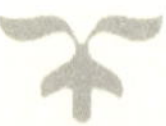

## SLOW COOKER PULLED PORK

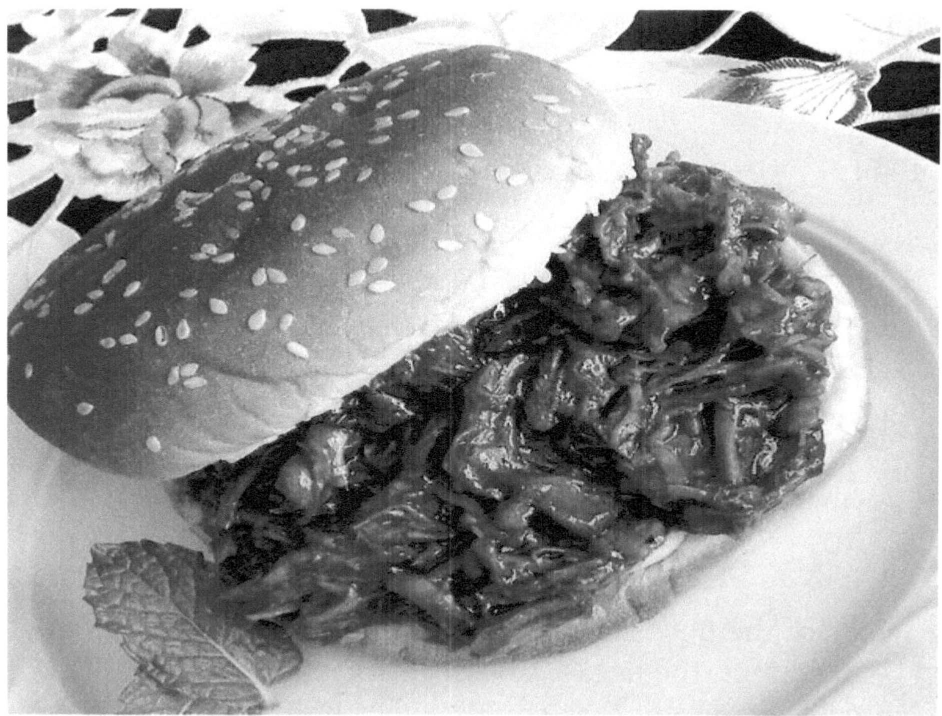

Pork simmered in root beer makes all the difference. Topped with your favorite BBQ sauce, it's sure to bring rave reviews.

## INGREDIENTS

- 1 (2 pound) pork tenderloin
- 1 (12 fluid ounce) can or bottle root beer
- 1 (18 ounce) bottle your favorite barbecue sauce

- 8 hamburger buns, split and lightly toasted

# DIRECTIONS

Prep
10 m

Cook
7 hr

Ready In
7 hr 10 m

Servings
8

- Place the pork tenderloin in a slow cooker; pour the root beer over the meat. Cover and cook on low until well cooked and the pork shreds easily, 6 to 7 hours. Note: the actual length of time may vary according to individual slow cooker. Drain well. Stir in barbecue sauce. Serve over hamburger buns.

# NUTRITION FACTS

Per Serving: 335 calories; 5 g total fat; 49 mg cholesterol; 990 mg sodium. 49.4 g carbohydrates; 21.2 g protein;

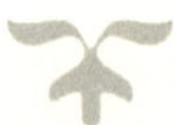

# MAPLE SALMON

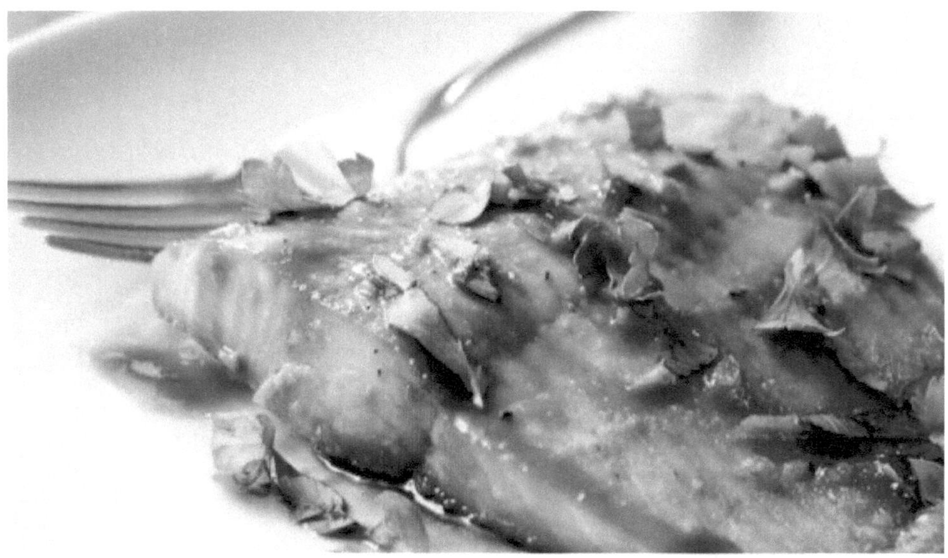

"This is the best and most delicious salmon recipe, and very easy to prepare. I love maple in everything and put this together one night.

## INGREDIENTS

- 1/4 cup maple syrup
- 2 tablespoons soy sauce
- 1 clove garlic, minced
- 1/4 teaspoon garlic salt
- 1/8 teaspoon ground black pepper
- 1 pound salmon

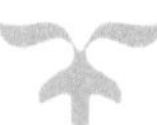

# DIRECTIONS

Prep
10 m

Cook
20 m

Ready In
1 h

Servings
4

- In a small bowl, mix the maple syrup, soy sauce, garlic, garlic salt, and pepper.
- Place salmon in a shallow glass baking dish, and coat with the maple syrup mixture. Cover the dish, and marinate salmon in the refrigerator 30 minutes, turning once.
- Preheat oven to 400 degrees F (200 degrees C).
- Place the baking dish in the preheated oven, and bake salmon uncovered 20 minutes, or until easily flaked with a fork.

# NUTRITION FACTS

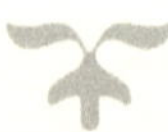

Per Serving: 265 calories; 12.4 g fat; 14.1 g carbohydrates; 23.2 g protein; 67 mg cholesterol; 633 mg sodium.

# SALSA CHICKEN

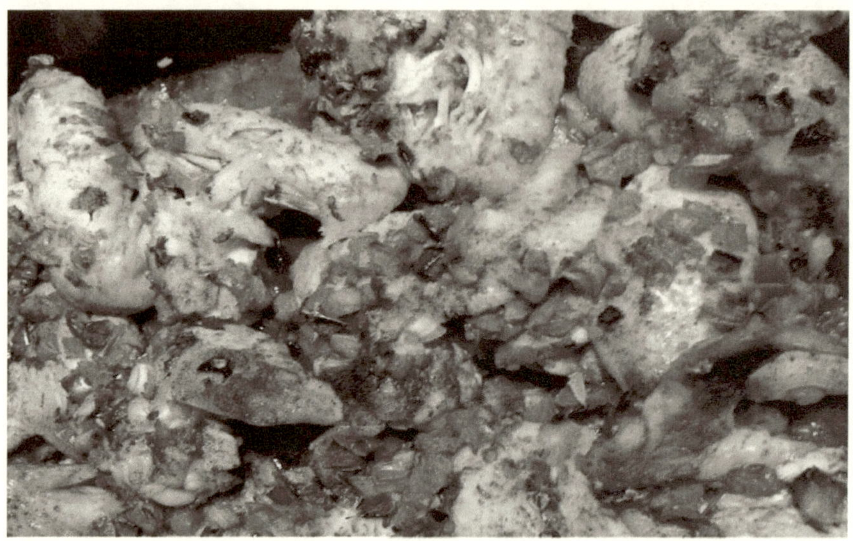

Boneless, skinless chicken breasts stay juicy baked in this beautiful Homemade Restaurant Style Salsa, getting all the flavors from tomatoes, onions, jalapenos, and garlic.

## INGREDIENTS

- 4 skinless, boneless chicken breast halves
- 4 teaspoons taco seasoning mix
- 1 cup salsa
- 1 cup shredded Cheddar cheese
- 2 tablespoons sour cream (optional)

# DIRECTIONS

Prep
5 m

Cook
40 m

Ready In
45 m

Servings
4

- Preheat oven to 375 degrees F (190 degrees C)

- Place chicken breasts in a lightly greased 9x13 inch baking dish. Sprinkle taco seasoning on both sides of chicken breasts, and pour salsa over all.

- Bake at 375 degrees F (190 degrees C) for 25 to 35 minutes, or until chicken is tender and juicy and its juices run clear.

- Sprinkle chicken evenly with cheese, and continue baking for an additional 3 to 5 minutes, or until cheese is melted and bubbly. Top with sour cream if desired, and serve.

# NUTRITION FACTS

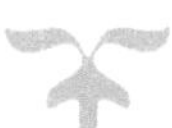

Per Serving: 287 calories; 12.4 g total fat; 101 mg cholesterol; 863 mg sodium. 6.8 g carbohydrates; 35.5 g protein;

# ZESTY SLOW COOKER CHICKEN BARBECUE

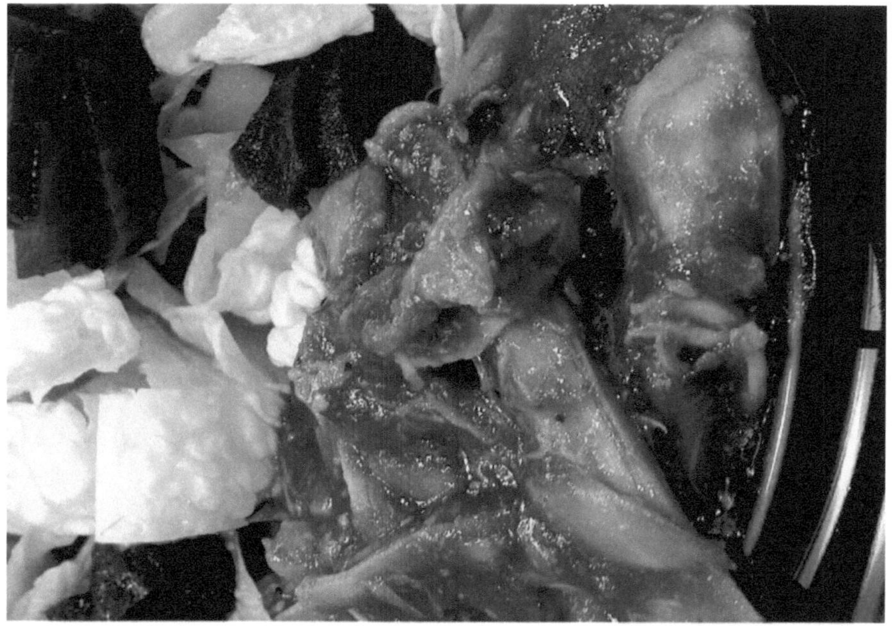

Use your slow cooker to prepare this great twist on basic barbecue chicken. Throw the chicken breasts in frozen, and serve with baked potatoes.

## INGREDIENTS

- 6 frozen skinless, boneless chicken breast halves

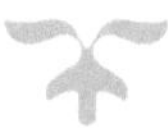

- 1 (12 ounce) bottle barbeque sauce
- ½ cup Italian salad dressing
- ¼ cup brown sugar
- 2 tablespoons Worcestershire sauce

# DIRECTIONS

Prep
10 m

Cook
4 hr

Ready In
4 hr 10 m

Servings
6

- Place chicken in a slow cooker. In a bowl, mix the barbecue sauce, Italian salad dressing, brown sugar, and Worcestershire sauce. Pour over the chicken.

- Cover, and cook 3 to 4 hours on High or 6 to 8 hours on Low.

# NUTRITION FACTS

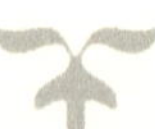

Per Serving: 300 calories; 8.1 g total fat; 61 mg cholesterol; 1058 mg sodium. 32.4 g carbohydrates; 23 g protein;

## LOW-CAL CHICKEN

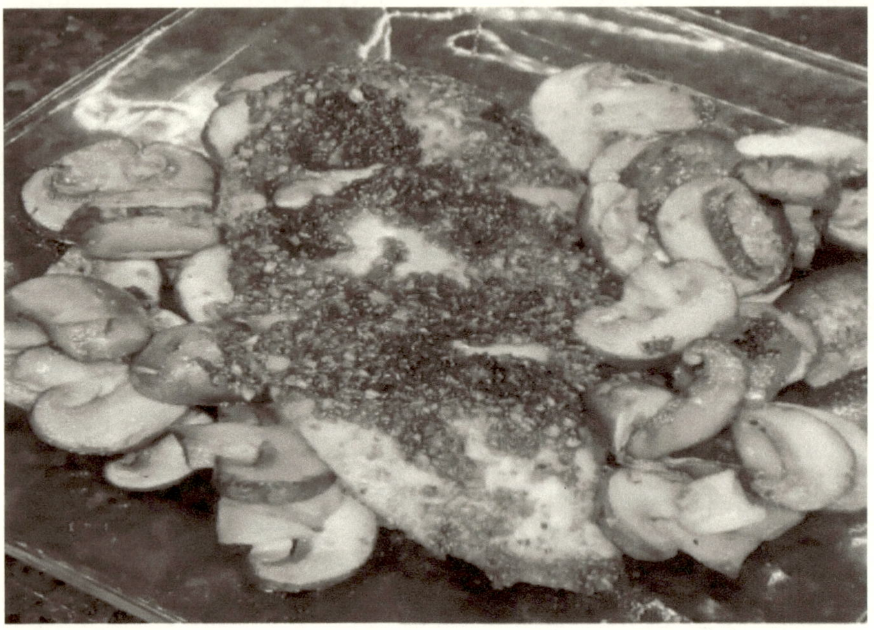

Use your slow cooker to prepare this great twist on basic barbecue chicken. Throw the chicken breasts in frozen, and serve with baked potatoes.

## INGREDIENTS

- 4 (4 ounce) skinless, boneless chicken breast halves
- 1 ½ tablespoons minced onion
- 2 tablespoons crushed garlic
- 1 ½ teaspoons poultry seasoning

- ¼ cup soy sauce
- 2 teaspoons artificial sweetener

# DIRECTIONS

Servings
4

- Preheat oven to 425 degrees F (220 degrees C).

- Place chicken in a 9x13 inch baking dish; sprinkle with onion, garlic, seasoning, soy sauce and sweetener.

- Place foil over pan and bake for one hour at 425 degrees F (220 degrees C). It's ready to serve!

# NUTRITION FACTS

Per Serving: 142 calories; 2.4 g total fat; 59 mg cholesterol; 952 mg sodium. 3.3 g carbohydrates; 25.8 g protein;

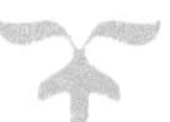

# BBQ PORK FOR SANDWICHES

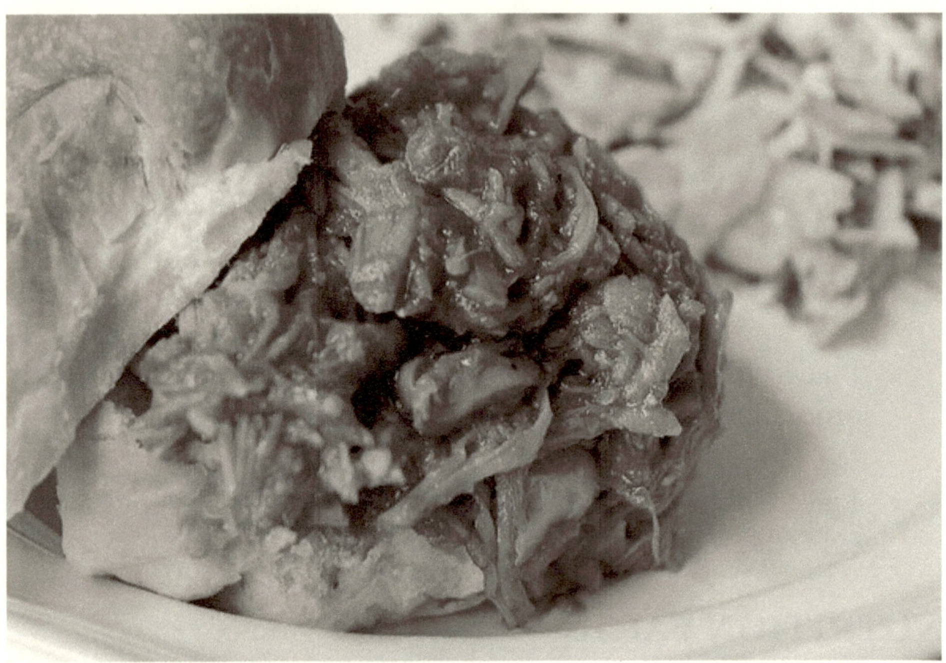

This is so easy and very tasty. Serve on buns with French fries or potato chips.

## INGREDIENTS

- 1 (14 ounce) can beef broth
- 3 pounds boneless pork ribs
- 1 (18 ounce) bottle barbeque sauce

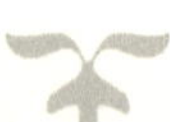

# DIRECTIONS

Prep
15 m

Cook
4 hr  30 m

Ready In
4 hr 45 m

Servings
12

- Pour can of beef broth into slow cooker, and add boneless pork ribs. Cook on High heat for 4 hours, or until meat shreds easily. Remove meat, and shred with two forks. It will seem that it's not working right away, but it will.

- Preheat oven to 350 degrees F (175 degrees C). Transfer the shredded pork to a Dutch oven or iron skillet, and stir in barbeque sauce.

- Bake in the preheated oven for 30 minutes, or until heated through.

# NUTRITION FACTS

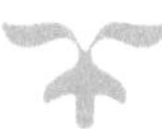

Per Serving: 355 calories; 18.1 g total fat; 83 mg cholesterol; 623 mg sodium. 15.2 g carbohydrates; 30.2 g protein;

## GARLIC CHICKEN LIVERS

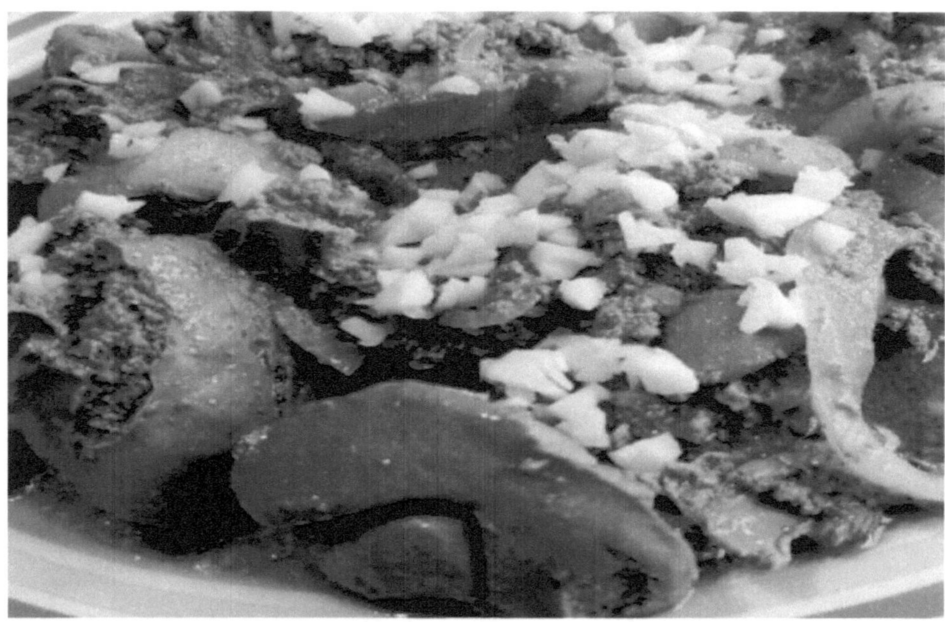

This is the ultimate garlic chicken liver recipe. Simple, quick, minimal ingredients, and low in carbs! The lemon, garlic, and liver flavors blend together to to make a surprisingly mild gourmet dish.

# INGREDIENTS

- 1 pound chicken livers - rinsed, trimmed, and patted dry
- 1 ½ tablespoons olive oil
- 2 teaspoons lemon juice
- ½ teaspoon salt, or to taste

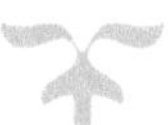

- 6 cloves garlic, minced

# DIRECTIONS

Prep
10 m

Cook
5 m

Ready In
15 m

Servings
4

- Heat a skillet over medium heat. Cook and stir livers in the hot skillet until cooked through, 3 to 5 minutes. Add olive oil, lemon juice, and salt to livers; gently stir until mixed. Remove skillet from heat and sprinkle garlic over livers.

## NUTRITION FACTS

Per Serving: 174 calories; 9.8 g total fat; 410 mg cholesterol; 347 mg sodium. 2.4 g carbohydrates; 18.1 g protein;

# GARLIC PRIME RIB

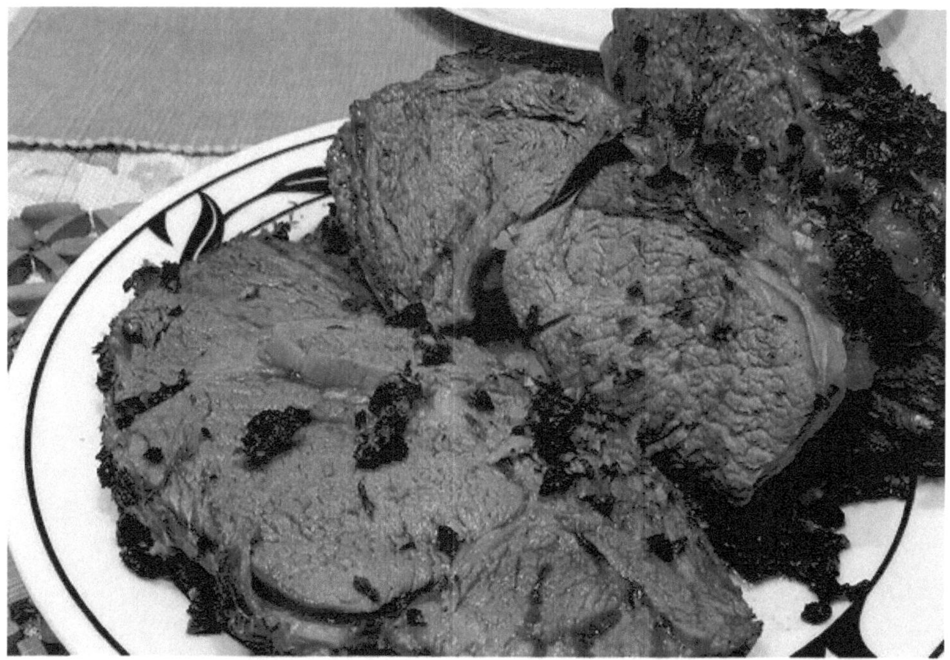

Quick and easy marinade and so tasty, I was trusted with this recipe but I can't keep it to myself!

## INGREDIENTS

- 1 (10 pound) prime rib roast
- 10 cloves garlic, minced
- 2 tablespoons olive oil
- 2 teaspoons salt

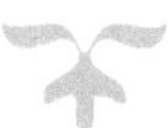

- 2 teaspoons ground black pepper
- 2 teaspoons dried thyme

# DIRECTIONS

Prep
10 m

Cook
1 hr 30 m

Ready In
1 hr 40 m

Servings
15

- Place the roast in a roasting pan with the fatty side up. In a small bowl, mix together the garlic, olive oil, salt, pepper and thyme. Spread the mixture over the fatty layer of the roast, and let the roast sit out until it is at room temperature, no longer than 1 hour.

- Preheat the oven to 500 degrees F (260 degrees C).

- Bake the roast for 20 minutes in the preheated oven, then reduce the temperature to 325 degrees F (165 degrees C), and continue roasting for an additional 60 to 75 minutes.

The internal temperature of the roast should be at 135 degrees F (57 degrees C) for medium rare.

- Allow the roast to rest for 10 or 15 minutes before carving so the meat can retain its juices.

## NUTRITION FACTS

Per Serving: 562 calories; 48 g total fat; 113 mg cholesterol; 395 mg sodium. 1 g carbohydrates; 29.6 g protein;

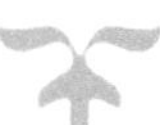

# BBQ RIBS

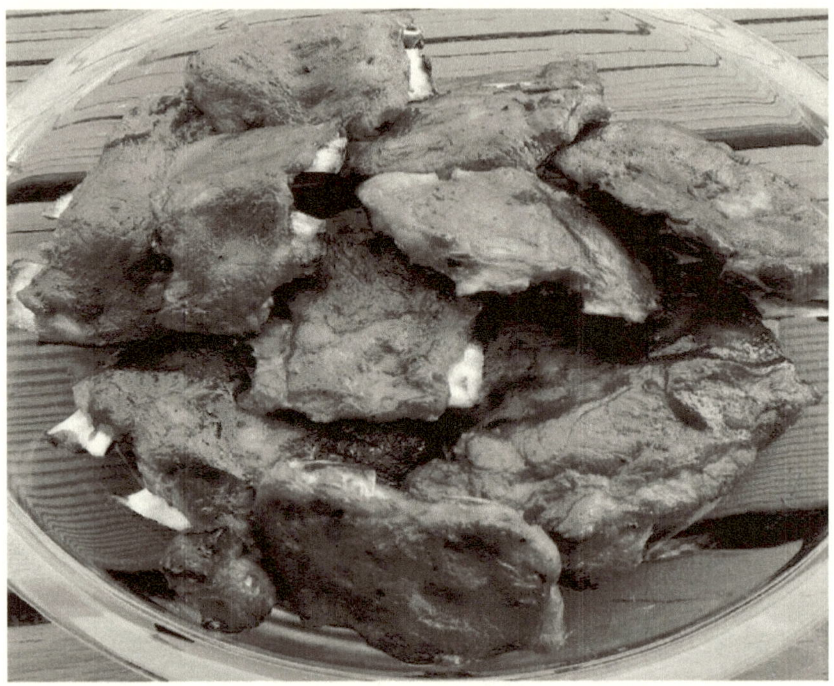

Country-style ribs are cut from the loin, one of the leanest areas of pork. These ribs are seasoned, boiled until tender, then baked with your favorite barbeque sauce. That's it! Back to simplicity, back to the country life. Sigh.

## INGREDIENTS

- 2 ½ pounds country style pork ribs
- 1 tablespoon garlic powder

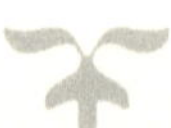

- 1 teaspoon ground black pepper
- 2 tablespoons salt
- 1 cup barbeque sauce

# DIRECTIONS

Prep
30 m

Cook
1 hr 30 m

Ready In
2 hr

Servings
4

- Place ribs in a large pot with enough water to cover. Season with garlic powder, black pepper and salt. Bring water to a boil, and cook ribs until tender.

- Preheat oven to 325 degrees F (165 degrees C).

- Remove ribs from pot, and place them in a 9x13 inch baking dish. Pour barbeque sauce over ribs. Cover dish with aluminum foil, and bake in the preheated oven for 1 to

1 1/2 hours, or until internal temperature of pork has reached 160 degrees F (70 degrees C).

## NUTRITION FACTS

Per Serving: 441 calories; 22.2 g total fat; 128 mg cholesterol; 4260 mg sodium. 24.5 g carbohydrates; 33.3 g protein;

## JUICY ROASTED CHICKEN

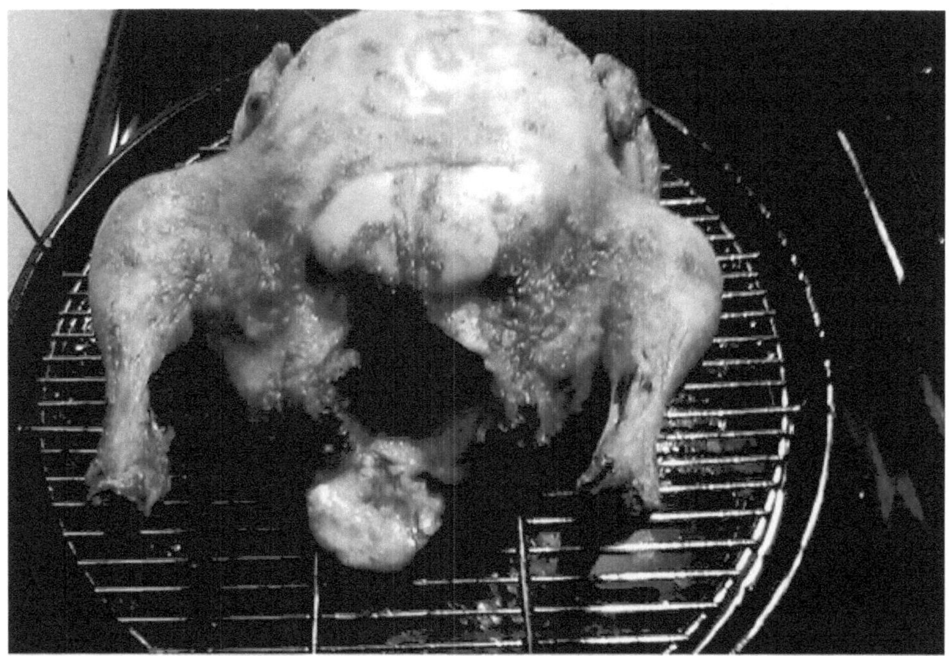

A juicy, crispy roast chicken with vegetables is one recipe every home cook can and should easily master.

## INGREDIENTS

- 1 (3 pound) whole chicken, giblets removed
- salt and black pepper to taste
- 1 tablespoon onion powder, or to taste
- ½ cup margarine, divided
- 1 stalk celery, leaves removed

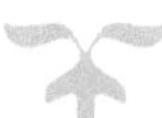

# DIRECTIONS

Prep
30 m

Cook
1 hr 15 m

Ready In
1 hr 45 m

Servings
6

- Preheat oven to 350 degrees F (175 degrees C).

- Place chicken in a roasting pan, and season generously inside and out with salt and pepper. Sprinkle inside and out with onion powder. Place 3 tablespoons margarine in the chicken cavity. Arrange dollops of the remaining margarine around the chicken's exterior. Cut the celery into 3 or 4 pieces, and place in the chicken cavity.

- Bake uncovered 1 hour and 15 minutes in the preheated oven, to a minimum internal temperature of 180 degrees F (82 degrees C). Remove from heat, and baste with melted margarine and drippings. Cover with aluminum foil, and allow to rest about 30 minutes before serving.

## NUTRITION FACTS

Per Serving: 423 calories; 32.1 g total fat; 97 mg cholesterol; 662 mg sodium. 1.2 g carbohydrates; 30.9 g protein;

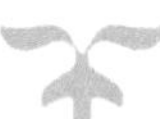

# FOOLPROOF RIB ROAST

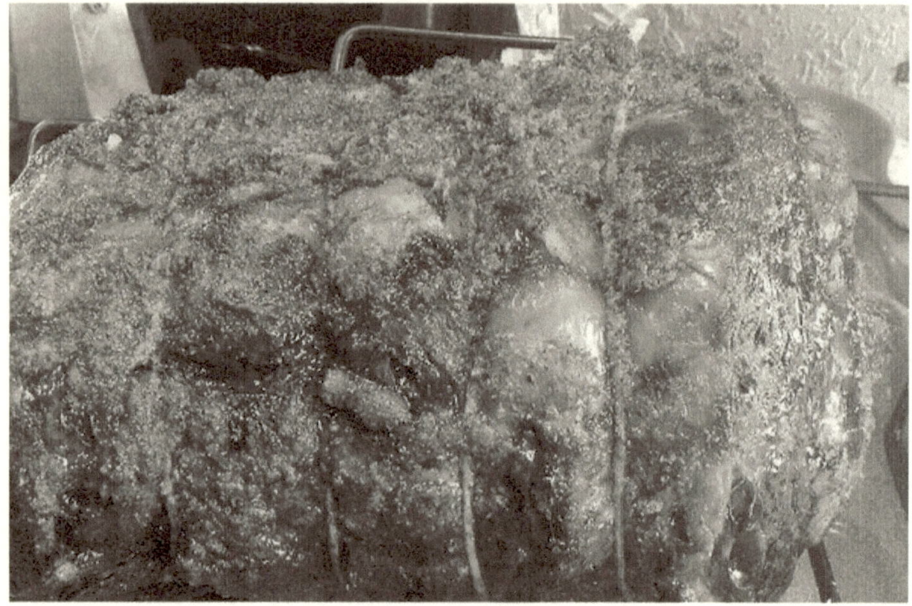

It turned out PERFECT. Rib Roast can be expensive, so this is a total splurge or special occasion dish. Enjoy.

## INGREDIENTS

- 1 (5 pound) standing beef rib roast
- 2 teaspoons salt
- 1 teaspoon ground black pepper
- 1 teaspoon garlic powder

# DIRECTIONS

Prep
5 m

Cook
5 hr

Ready In
5 hr 5 m

Servings
6

- Allow roast to stand at room temperature for at least 1 hour.

- Preheat the oven to 375 degrees F (190 degrees C). Combine the salt, pepper and garlic powder in a small cup. Place the roast on a rack in a roasting pan so that the fatty side is up and the rib side is on the bottom. Rub the seasoning onto the roast.

- Roast for 1 hour in the preheated oven. Turn the oven off and leave the roast inside. Do not open the door. Leave it in there for 3 hours. 30 to 40 minutes before serving, turn the oven back on at 375 degrees F (190 degrees C) to reheat the roast. The internal temperature should be at least 145

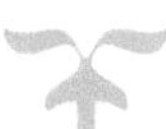

degrees F (62 degrees C). Remove from the oven and let rest for 10 minutes before carving into servings.

## NUTRITION FACTS

Per Serving: 576 calories; 46.2 g total fat; 137 mg cholesterol; 880 mg sodium. 0.6 g carbohydrates; 37 g protein;

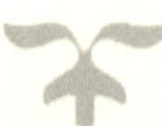

# PUFFS

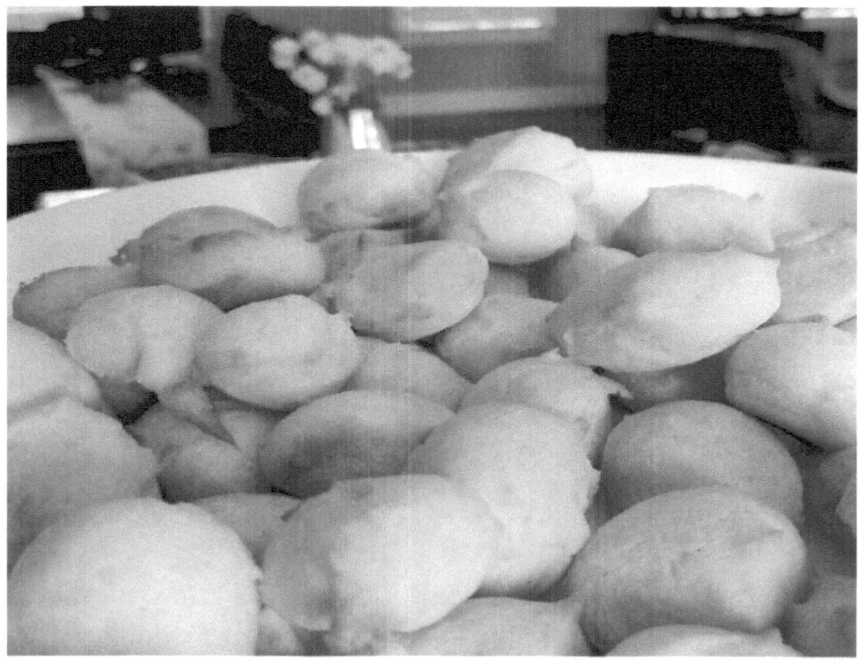

Puffs that you put tuna, ham, chicken, shrimp, or egg salads. This is a wonderful basic recipe that you can build on and create sweet or savory dishes. Stuff them with vanilla ice cream and top with chocolate sauce. Voila, a fabulous dessert that looks like you spent hours on, but you didn't!

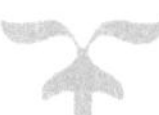

# INGREDIENTS

- ¼ cup butter
- ½ cup water
- ½ cup all-purpose flour
- 2 eggs

# DIRECTIONS

Servings
20

- Preheat oven to 375 degrees F (190 degrees C). Grease a cookie sheet. Set aside.

- In a medium saucepan heat butter and water over medium heat until butter melts. Fold in flour all at once, and stir vigorously until a ball forms in the center of the pan. Remove from heat and let stand for 5 minutes.

- Add eggs, one at a time, and beat until fully blended. Mix should be very stiff. Drop by 1/2 to 3/4 teaspoon onto prepared cookie sheet.

- Bake for 30 to 40 minutes, or until the moisture disappears. Cool and slit a small opening on one side and stuff with desired filling.

# NUTRITION FACTS

Per Serving: 39 calories; 2.8 g total fat; 25 mg cholesterol; 23 mg sodium. 2.4 g carbohydrates; 1 g protein

# CREAM DILL SAUCE

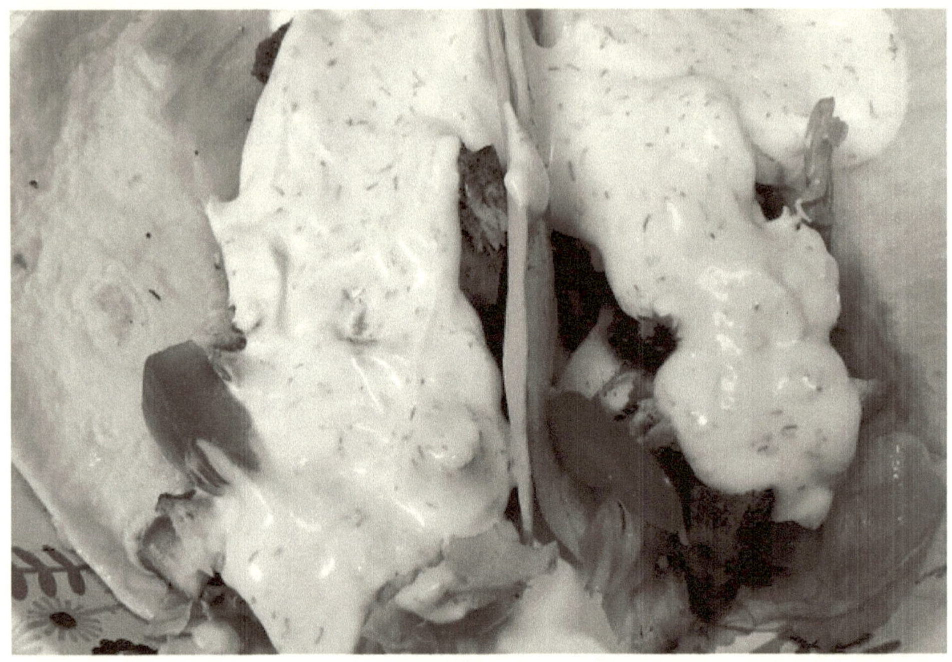

This is a tangy sauce of sour cream, mayonnaise, green onions, dill weed and lemon juice. Serve over potatoes, or as a dip for vegetables.

## INGREDIENTS

- 1 cup sour cream
- ¾ cup mayonnaise
- 2 tablespoons finely chopped green onions
- 2 teaspoons dried dill weed

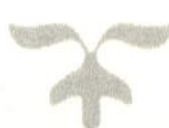

- 2 tablespoons lemon juice

## DIRECTIONS

Prep
10 m

Cook
1 hr

Ready In
1 hr 10 m

Servings
8

- In a medium bowl combine sour cream, mayonnaise, green onions, dill and lemon juice. Mix well and chill for at least 1 hour.

## NUTRITION FACTS

Per Serving: 212 calories; 22.4 g total fat; 20 mg cholesterol; 133 mg sodium. 2.5 g carbohydrates; 1.2 g protein;

# SHRIMP SCAMPI BAKE

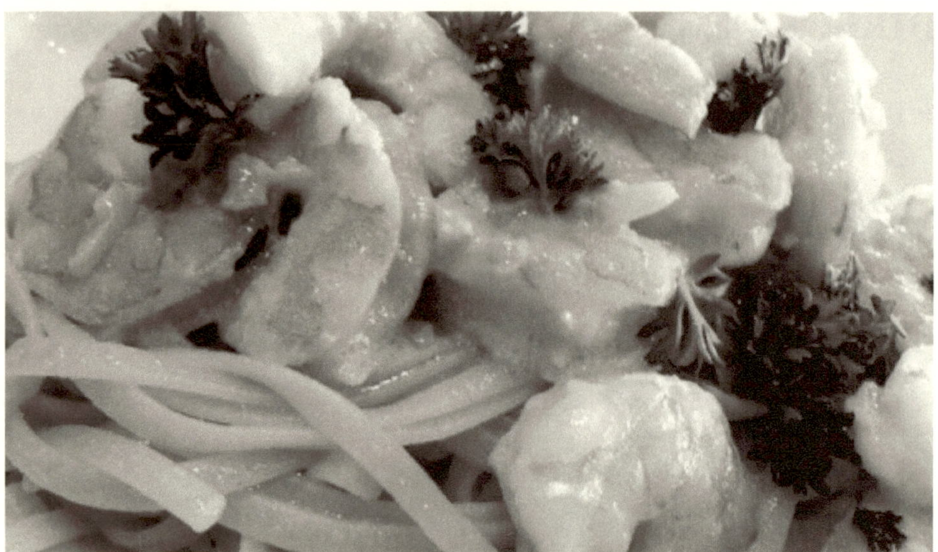

"Easy version of this classic with the wonderful 'zip' of Dijon-style mustard."

## INGREDIENTS

- 1 cup butter
- 2 tablespoons prepared Dijon-style mustard
- 1 tablespoon fresh lemon juice
- 1 tablespoon chopped garlic
- 1 tablespoon chopped fresh parsley
- 2 pounds medium raw shrimp, shelled, deveined, with tails attached

# DIRECTIONS

Prep
30 m

Cook
15 m

Ready In
45 m

Servings
6

- Preheat oven to 450 degrees F (230 degrees C).
- In a small saucepan over medium heat, combine the butter, mustard, lemon juice, garlic, and parsley. When the butter melts completely, remove from heat.
- Arrange shrimp in a shallow baking dish. Pour the butter mixture over the shrimp.
- Bake in preheated oven for 12 to 15 minutes or until the shrimp are pink and opaque.

# NUTRITION FACTS

Per Serving: 420 calories; 32.8 g fat; 1.8 g carbohydrates; 30 g protein; 320 mg cholesterol; 681 mg sodium.

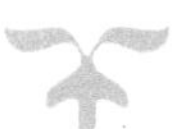

# MOCK SLIDERS

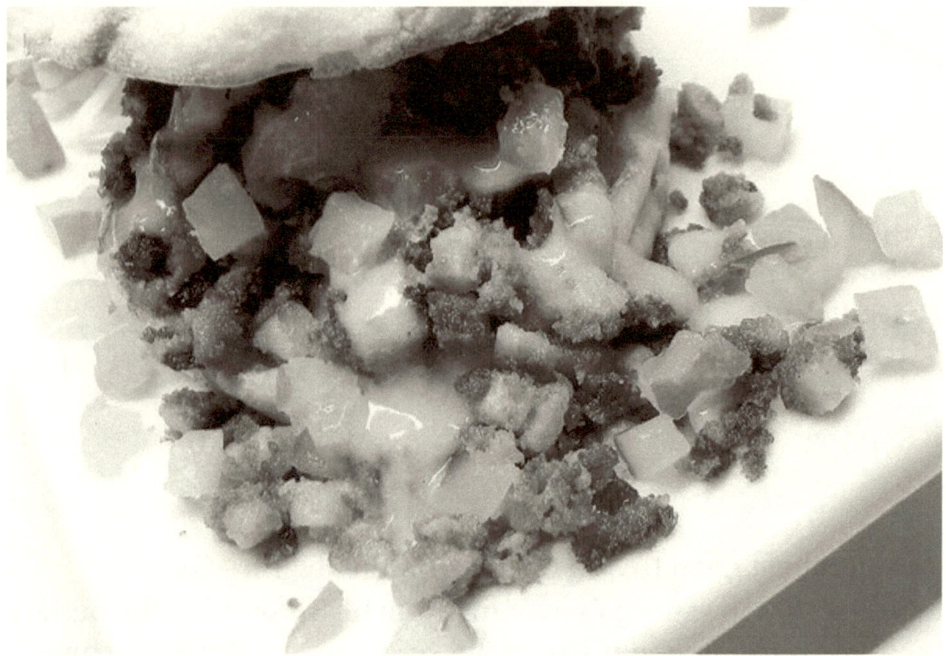

These will do when you can't get the real thing. Cocktail sandwiches are filled with a creamy, flavorful corned beef mixture and topped with a pickle.

## INGREDIENTS

- 1 (12 ounce) can corned beef, chopped
- 1 (8 ounce) container sour cream
- 1 (1 ounce) envelope dry onion soup mix

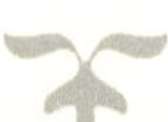

- 2 (8 ounce) packages dinner rolls
- 1 (16 ounce) jar dill pickle slices, drained

# DIRECTIONS

Prep
15 m

Cook
1 m

Ready In
16 m

Servings
24

- In a medium bowl, mix together corned beef, sour cream and dry onion soup mix.

- Cut rolls in half horizontally. Spread bottoms with the corned beef mixture. Replace tops.

- Microwave 30 to 45 seconds on high heat, until hot and moist. Top with dill pickle slices before serving.

# NUTRITION FACTS

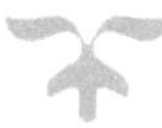

Per Serving: 62 calories; 4.1 g total fat; 16 mg cholesterol; 489 mg sodium. 1.9 g carbohydrates; 4.3 g protein;

# SARGE'S EZ PULLED PORK BBQ

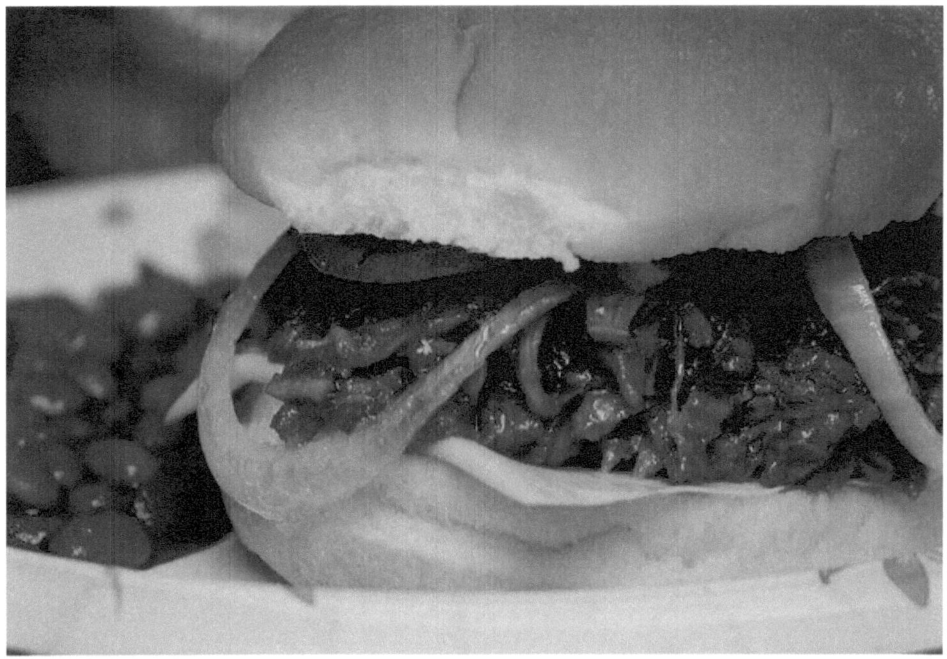

Too busy to cook? A slow cooker and a can of beef broth gets you started on this recipe. 'Low and slow' cooking gives you a roast that shreds with a fork. As an added bonus you get great stock for beef gravy as a by-product! Serve with your favorite BBQ sauce and plenty of coleslaw.

## INGREDIENTS

- 1 (5 pound) pork butt roast

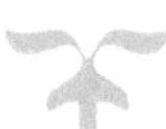

- salt and pepper to taste
- 1 (14 ounce) can beef broth
- ¼ cup brewed coffee

# DIRECTIONS

Prep
10 m

Cook
8 hr

Ready In
8 hr 10 m

Servings
10

- Cut roast in half. Rub each half with salt and pepper, and place in the slow cooker. Pour broth and coffee over the meat.

- Turn the slow cooker to Low, and cover. Cook for 6 to 8 hours, or until the roast is fork tender.

- Carefully remove the roast to a cutting board. Pull the meat off the bone with a fork. You may also chop it with a cleaver afterwards, if you like it really finely cut.

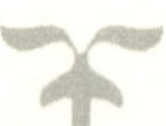

# NUTRITION FACTS

Per Serving: 270 calories; 18.8 g total fat; 85 mg cholesterol; 196 mg sodium. 0 g carbohydrates; 23.4 g protein;

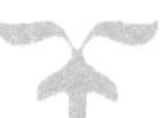

# FESTIVE ONIONS

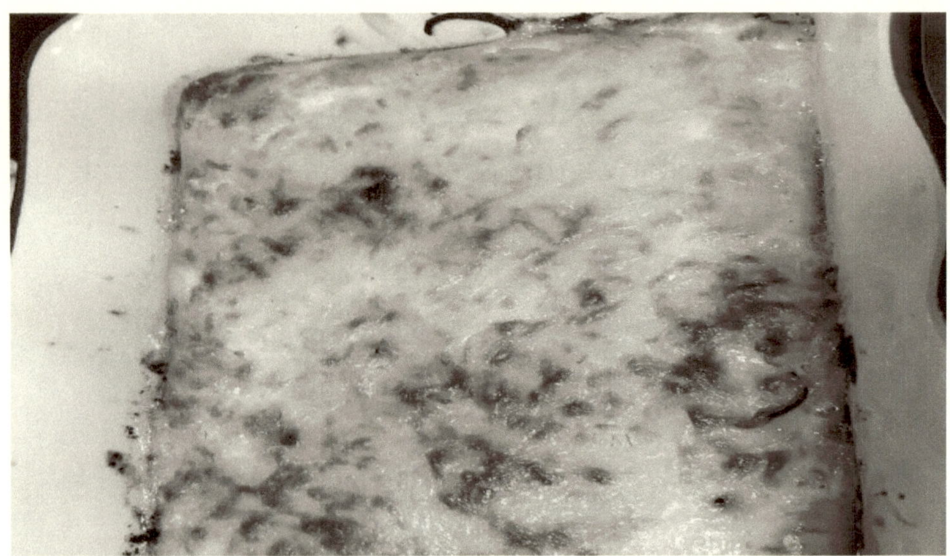

A simple to prepare, creamy onion dish.

## INGREDIENTS

- 4 cups sliced onion
- 5 tablespoons butter
- 1 cup cream
- salt to taste
- ground black pepper to taste
- ⅔ cup Parmesan cheese
- 2 eggs

# DIRECTIONS

Servings
7

- Saute onions in butter or margarine until transparent. Place in 2-quart baking dish.

- In a small bowl, beat eggs well. Stir in cream, and season with salt and pepper. Pour mixture over onions, and sprinkle cheese.

- Bake, uncovered, at 425 degrees F (220 degrees C) for 15 to 20 minutes.

# NUTRITION FACTS

Per Serving: 270 calories; 24.5 g total fat; 128 mg cholesterol; 210 mg sodium. 7.5 g carbohydrates; 6.2 g protein;

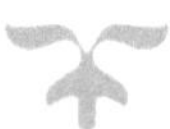

# CHICKEN GIZZARDS

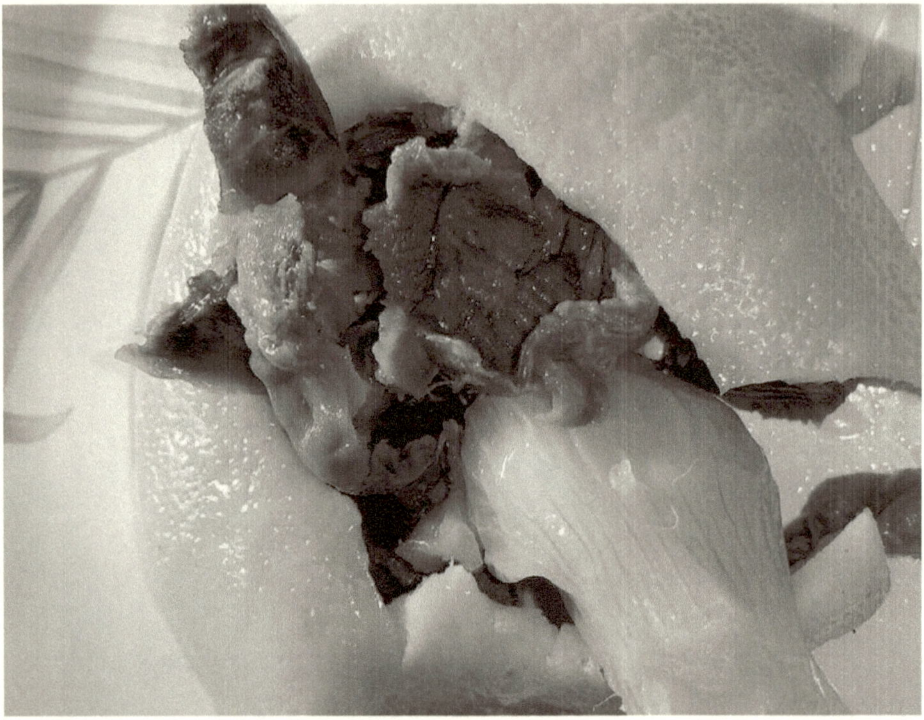

A simple to prepare, creamy onion dish.

## INGREDIENTS

- 1 pound chicken gizzards
- ¼ cup butter
- salt and pepper to taste

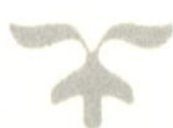

# DIRECTIONS

Prep
5 m

Cook
1 hr 45 m

Ready In
1 hr 50 m

Servings
4

- Place gizzards in a saucepan with enough water to cover by 1 inch. Bring to a boil over medium heat, cover, and cook for 1 1/2 hours. Drain and chop into bite size pieces.

- Melt butter in a large skillet over medium-high heat. Fry gizzards in butter for about 15 minutes. Season with salt and pepper to taste.

# NUTRITION FACTS

Per Serving: 195 calories; 13.2 g total fat; 267 mg cholesterol; 117 mg sodium. 0 g carbohydrates; 19.5 g protein;

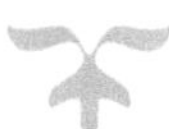

# MUSTARD CREAM SAUCE

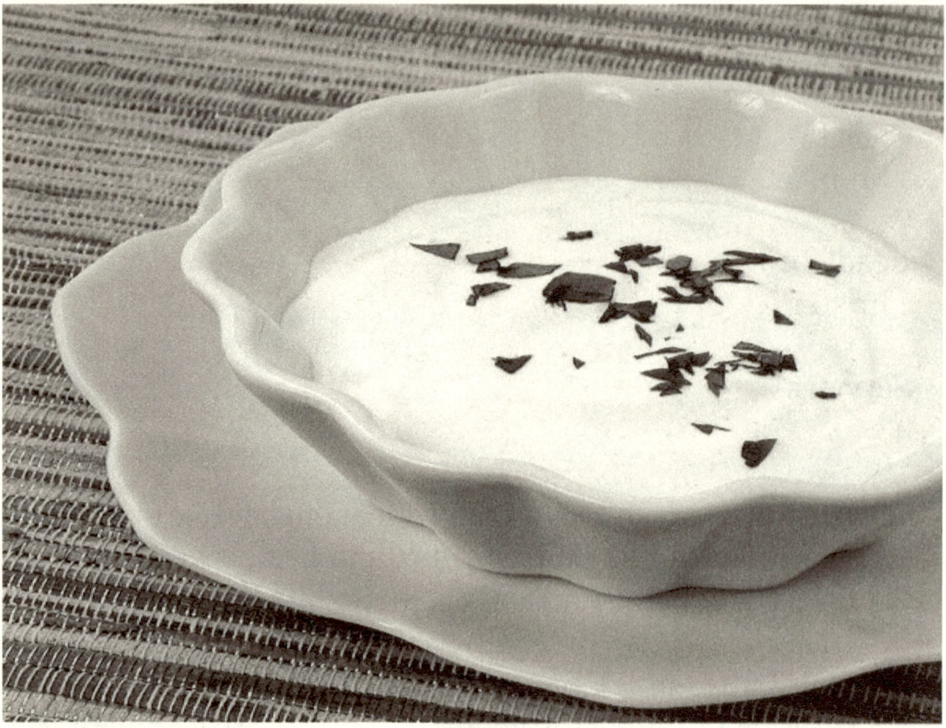

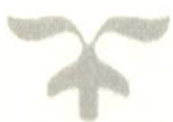

Here's a simple sauce that's perfect for crab cakes and other rich, savory appetizers. Dijon-style mustard is blended into a creamy mixture.

## INGREDIENTS

- ⅓ cup mayonnaise

- ¼ cup sour cream
- 1 tablespoon prepared Dijon-style mustard
- 1 tablespoon fresh lemon juice

# DIRECTIONS

Prep
5 m

Cook
0 m

Ready In
5 m

Servings
8

- In a medium bowl, whisk together mayonnaise, sour cream, Dijon-style mustard and lemon juice. Adjust amount of mustard to taste. Cover and chill in the refrigerator until serving.

## NUTRITION FACTS

Per Serving: 83 calories; 8.7 g total fat; 7 mg cholesterol; 102 mg sodium. 1.1 g carbohydrates; 0.3 g protein;

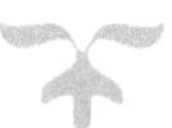

# SEARED CATFISH CREOLE

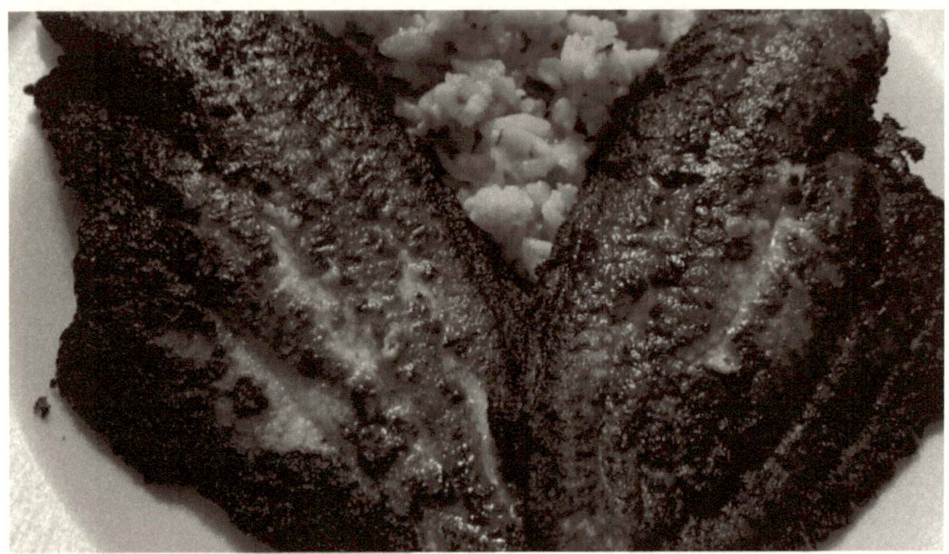

"A fast and easy but tasty and delicious catfish preparation with bite. You can vary the recipe by adding a layer of honey or using honey mustard. Also great with tuna!"

## INGREDIENTS

- 4 whole catfish, cleaned with head and tail removed
- 1/2 cup prepared yellow mustard
- 1/4 cup cracked black pepper
- 1/4 cup olive oil
- 1/4 cup butter

# DIRECTIONS

Prep
10 m

Cook
10 m

Ready In
20 m

Servings
8

- Pat the catfish dry, and spread a layer of mustard over the surface. Place the cracked pepper onto a plate, and press the coated catfish into the pepper so it is well covered.
- Heat the olive oil and butter in a large skillet over medium-high heat. Fry the catfish for 3 to 5 minutes on each side, or until fish flakes with a fork.

# NUTRITION FACTS

Per Serving: 331 calories; 23.9 g fat; 2.9 g carbohydrates; 25.9 g protein; 100 mg cholesterol; 326 mg sodium.

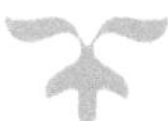

# KALUA PORK

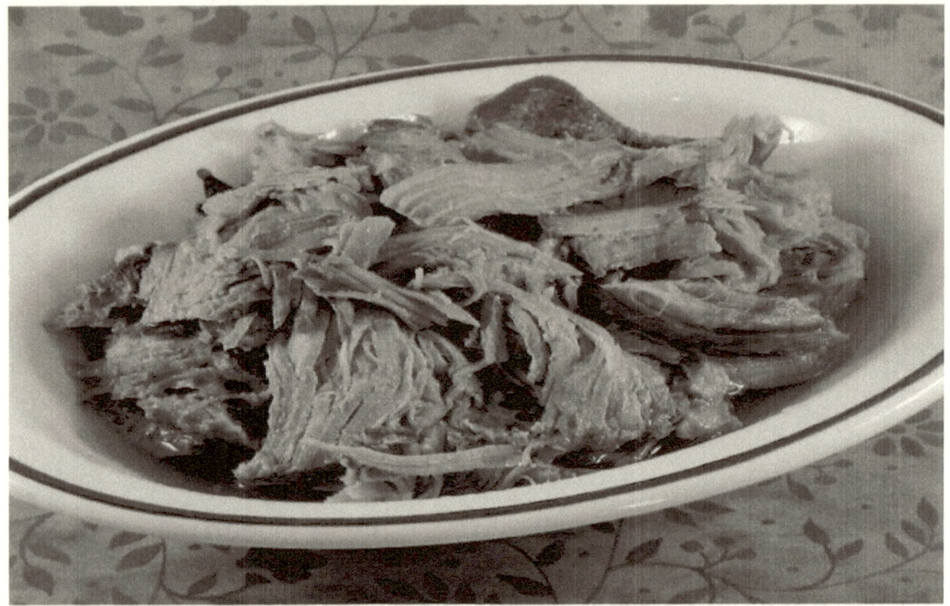

Savory pork butt with a smokey flavor. Any coarse salt can be used in place of the Hawaiian sea salt.

## INGREDIENTS

- 3 pounds pork butt roast
- 2 cups water
- 1 teaspoon liquid smoke flavoring
- ¼ cup Hawaiian sea salt

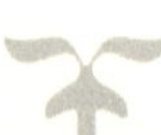

# DIRECTIONS

Prep
10 m

Cook
3 hr 10 m

Ready In
3 hr 20 m

Servings
6

- Preheat oven to 400 degrees F (200 degrees C).

- Place pork fat-side up in a roasting pan or deep casserole dish. Combine water and liquid smoke; pour over meat. Sprinkle with salt. Cover and roast in a preheated oven for three hours. Remove from pan and shred.

## NUTRITION FACTS

Per Serving: 264 calories; 17.2 g total fat; 94 mg cholesterol; 4960 mg sodium. 0 g carbohydrates; 25.4 g protein;

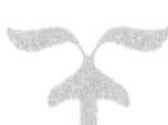

# SOFT SPREAD BUTTER

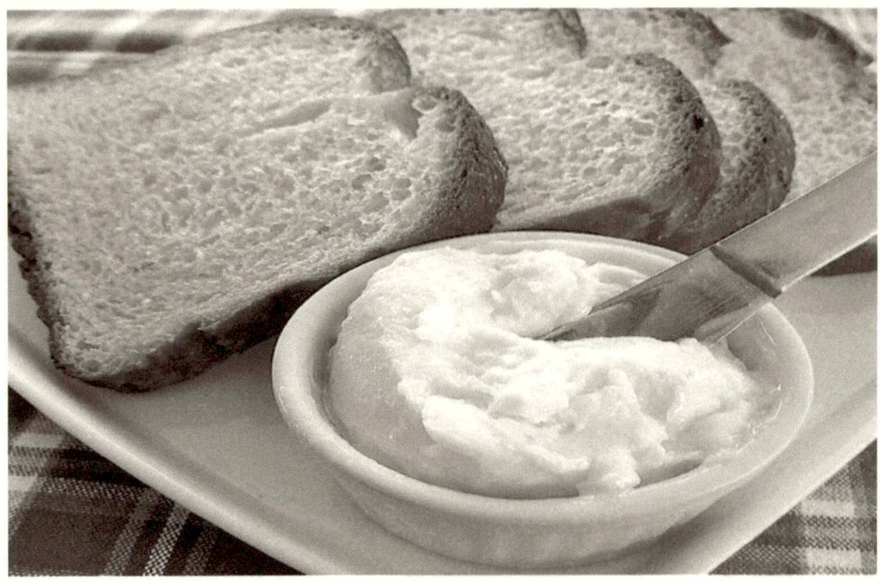

This is a homemade margarine or soft spread 'butter'. While it is not lower in calorie, it has a higher ratio of unsaturated to saturated fat than butter, and unlike margarine, it contains no trans fat. Create a flavored butter by adding garlic or cinnamon, or anything you chose!

## INGREDIENTS

- 1 cup butter, softened
- 1 ¼ cups canola oil

# DIRECTIONS

Prep
20 m

Ready In
3 hr 20 m

Servings
36

- In a lidded, plastic storage container stir butter until it has a smooth, frosting-like consistency.

- Slowly, one tablespoon at a time, stir in the first 1/2 cup of oil; mix until smooth. Stir in the remaining oil a little more quickly, mixing well.

- Refrigerate for 3 hours, or until set.

- Store in refrigerator. If the 'butter' melts after being left out, refrigerate to restore solidified quality.

# NUTRITION FACTS

Per Serving: 114 calories; 12.9 g total fat; 14 mg cholesterol; 36 mg sodium. 0 g carbohydrates; 0.1 g protein;

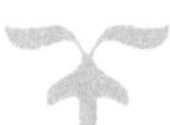

# CHICKEN ON A STICK

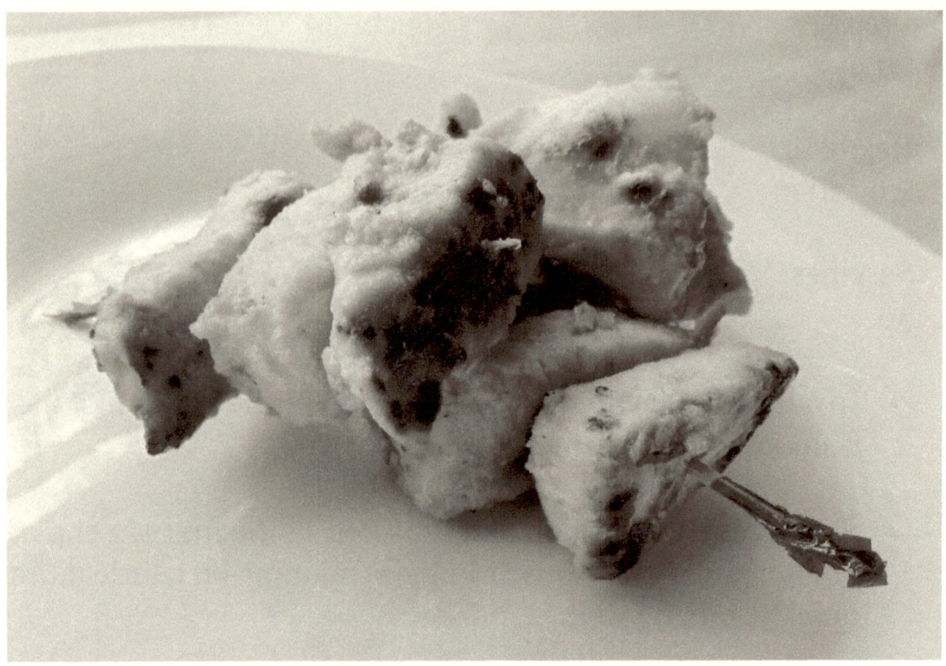

Easy recipe for marinated chicken breast cooked on skewers on the grill. These are so simple, and your family will love them!

## INGREDIENTS

- 4 skinless, boneless chicken breast halves
- 1 teaspoon meat tenderizer
- ½ cup Italian-style salad dressing

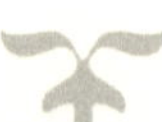

# DIRECTIONS

Prep
10 m

Cook
20 m

Ready In
1 hr 30 m

Servings
4

- Rinse chicken breasts and pat dry. Sprinkle with the meat tenderizer and place in a sealable plastic bag. Pour the dressing in the bag and turn the chicken to coat thoroughly. Seal and marinate in the refrigerator for 30 minutes to 1 hour.

- Preheat an outdoor grill for medium heat and lightly oil grate.

- Place the chicken onto skewers and grill over medium heat for 5 to 10 minutes per side. Chicken is done when its juices run clear.

# NUTRITION FACTS

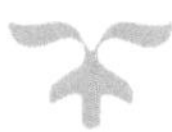

Per Serving: 218 calories; 9.8 g total fat; 68 mg cholesterol; 687 mg sodium. 3.1 g carbohydrates; 27.4 g protein;

# GREEN TURKEY AND CHEESE CASSEROLE

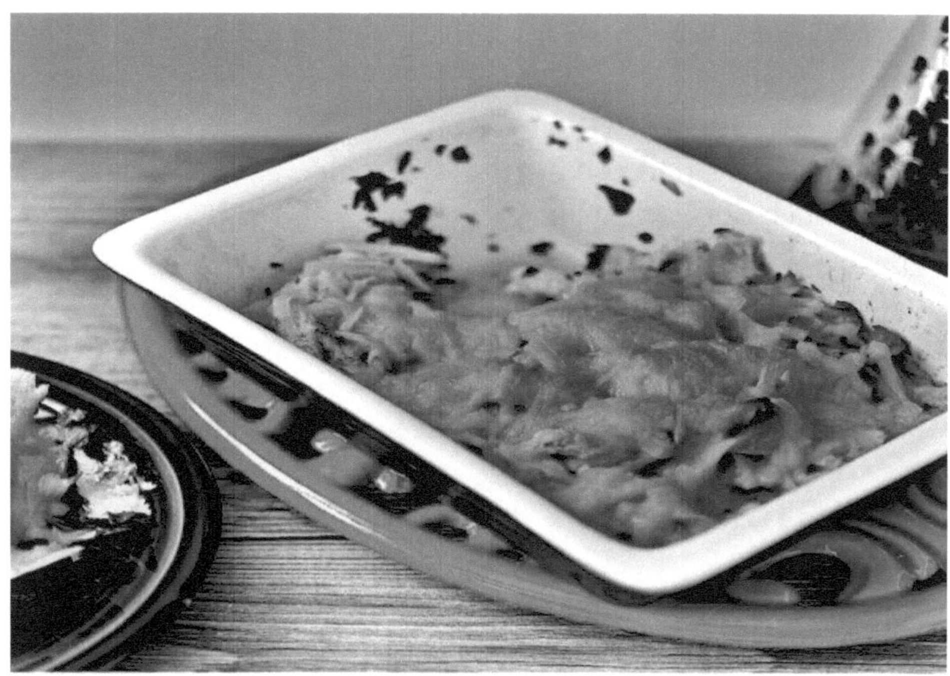

Easy recipe for marinated chicken breast cooked on skewers on the grill. These are so simple, and your family will love them!

## INGREDIENTS

- 1 pound spinach, rinsed and chopped
- 1 ½ cups cooked turkey, cubed
- 10 ounces shredded Cheddar cheese

# DIRECTIONS

Servings
5

- Preheat oven to 350 degrees F (175 degrees C). Grease one 10 inch casserole dish.

- Place the spinach in the prepared casserole dish. Top with the cubed turkey then with the grated cheese.

- Bake at 350 degrees F (175 degrees C) for 25 to 30 minutes.

# NUTRITION FACTS

Per Serving: 337 calories; 23.2 g total fat; 94 mg cholesterol; 452 mg sodium. 4 g carbohydrates; 28.5 g protein;

# MARINATED CHICKEN BARBECUE

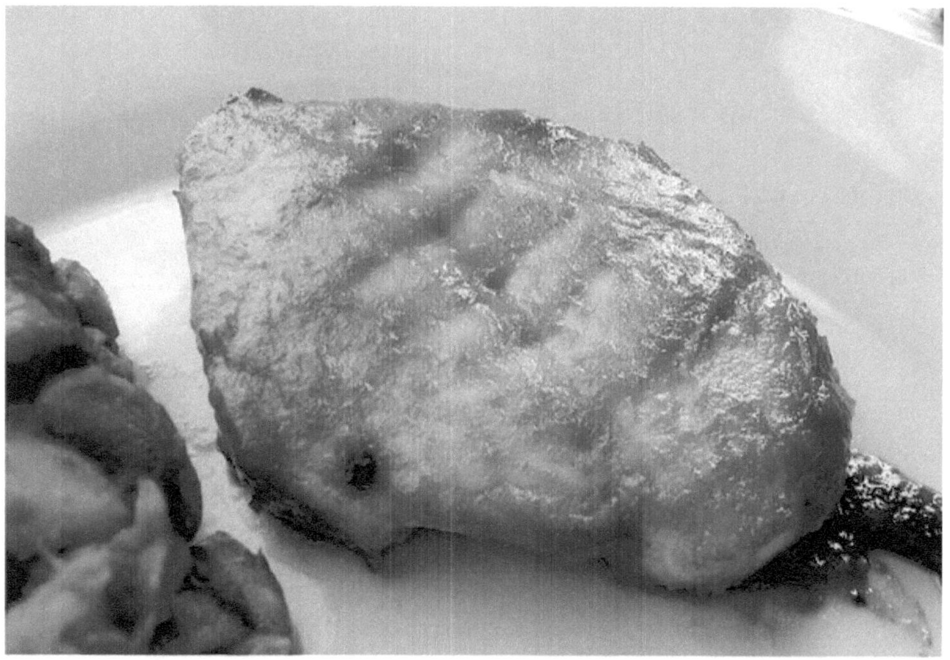

A quick and easy way to barbecue chicken using a marinade.

## INGREDIENTS

- 8 skinless, boneless chicken breasts
- 1 cup ketchup
- 2 tablespoons prepared horseradish
- ¼ cup lemon juice
- ½ cup vegetable oil

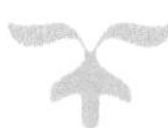

## DIRECTIONS

Servings
8

- Mix together ketchup, horseradish, lemon juice, and oil.

- Place chicken breasts in a dish, and pour marinade over. Refrigerate overnight.

- Bake at 350 degrees F (175 degrees C) for 45 minutes, basting every 15 minutes and turning once.

## NUTRITION FACTS

Per Serving: 284 calories; 15.3 g total fat; 68 mg cholesterol; 423 mg sodium. 8.6 g carbohydrates; 27.8 g protein;

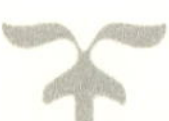

# SAVORY SPINACH CASSEROLE

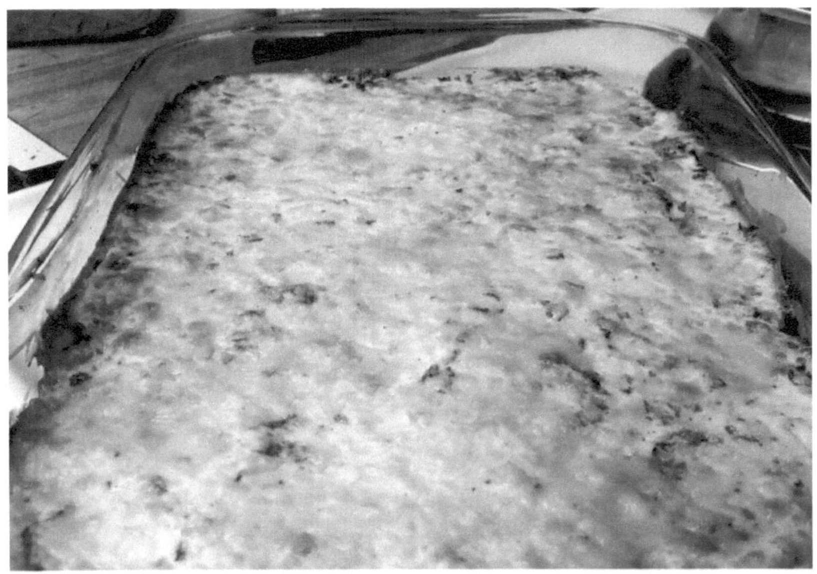

This cream cheese, spinach and Parmesan cheese dish is a very creamy and savory side dish!

## INGREDIENTS

- 1 (8 ounce) package cream cheese, softened
- ¼ cup milk
- 2 (10 ounce) packages frozen chopped spinach
- ⅓ cup grated Parmesan cheese

# DIRECTIONS

Prep
45 m

Cook
20 m

Ready In
1 hr 5 m

Servings
6

- Preheat oven to 350 degrees F (175 degrees C).

- In a mixing bowl, combine cream cheese and milk; mix until blended. Spoon spinach into 1-quart casserole, top with cream cheese mixture and sprinkle with Parmesan cheese.

- Bake in a preheated 350 degrees F (175 degrees C) oven for 20 minutes.

# NUTRITION FACTS

Per Serving: 180 calories; 15.1 g total fat; 47 mg cholesterol; 273 mg sodium. 5 g carbohydrates; 8 g protein;

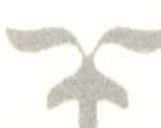

## HEALTHIER HOT LEGS

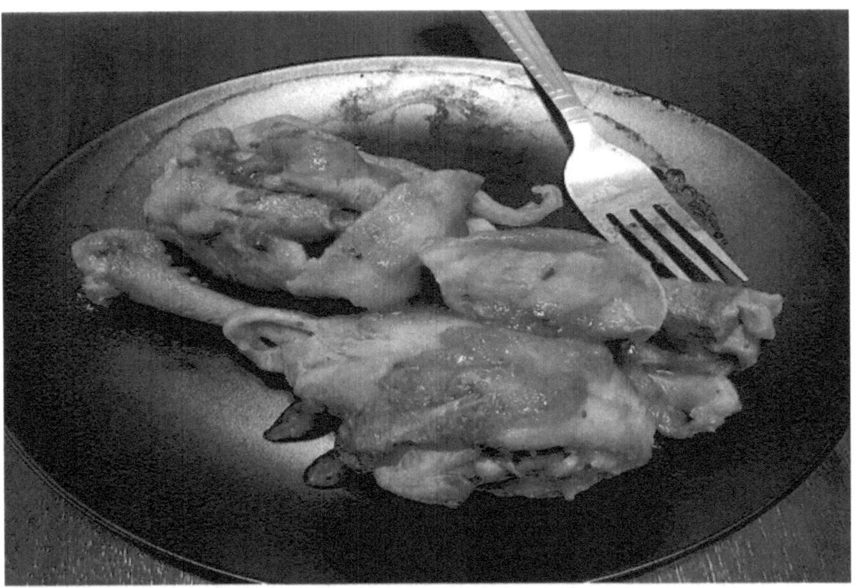

A tasty low carb and low fat substitute for Buffalo wings. Great for people with diabetes!

## INGREDIENTS

- 1 cup chili garlic sauce
- 1 (5 ounce) bottle Louisiana style hot sauce
- 2 tablespoons granular sucrolose sweetener (such as Splenda®)
- 1 tablespoon butter
- 12 skinless chicken drumsticks

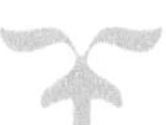

# DIRECTIONS

Prep
30 m

Cook
30 m

Ready In
1 hr

Servings
6

- In a medium bowl, stir together the chili garlic sauce, hot sauce and sweetener. Set aside.

- Melt butter in a large skillet over medium-high heat. Add the drumsticks, and cook until browned on the outside, turning as needed. Reduce heat to medium-low, and spoon sauce over the chicken to coat. Simmer, stirring occasionally, until chicken has cooked through and sauce is thick and sticky, about 20 minutes.

# NUTRITION FACTS

Per Serving: 187 calories; 6.3 g total fat; 101 mg cholesterol; 1964 mg sodium. 4.2 g carbohydrates; 25.9 g protein;

# GREEN CHICKEN

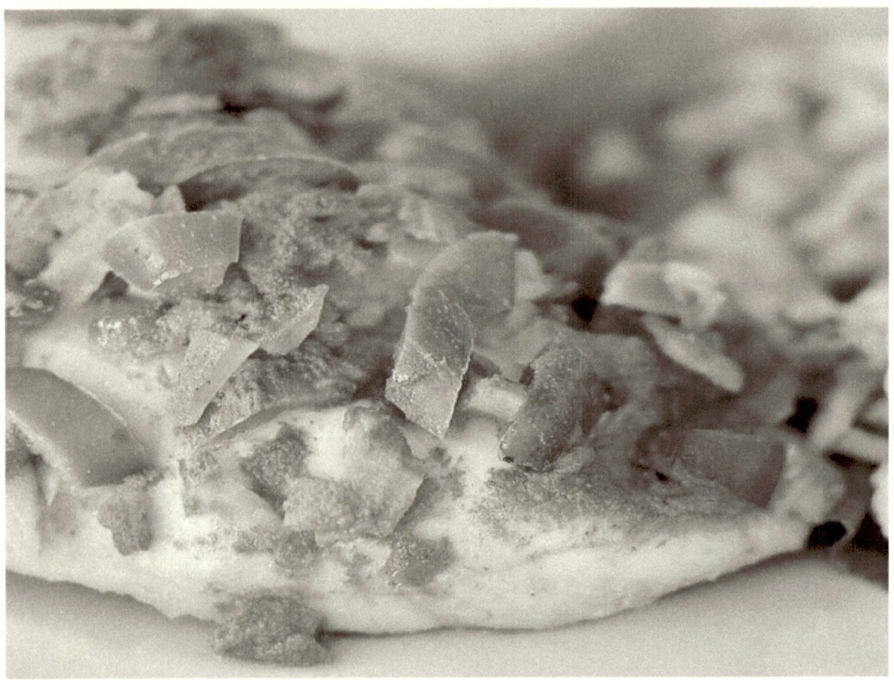

This is a fast and easy exotic chicken recipe made with chicken breasts. It gets it's green color from ground turmeric.

## INGREDIENTS

- 4 boneless, skinless chicken breast halves
- 1 onion, chopped
- 1 green bell pepper, seeded and chopped
- ¼ cup butter

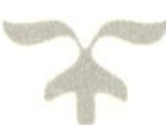

- 2 tablespoons ground turmeric
- salt and pepper to taste

# DIRECTIONS

Prep
10 m

Cook
1 hr

Ready In
1 hr 10 m

Servings
4

- Preheat the oven to 350 degrees F (175 degrees C).

- Place chicken breasts in a single layer in a 9x13 inch baking dish. Sprinkle the chopped onion and green pepper over the breasts. Place small pieces of butter around on the vegetables. Sprinkle turmeric powder evenly over the entire dish, and season with salt and pepper to taste. Cover the dish with a lid or aluminum foil.

- Bake for 45 to 60 minutes in the preheated oven, or until the chicken is no longer pink, and the juices run clear.

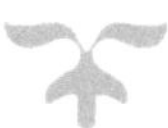

# NUTRITION FACTS

Per Serving: 262 calories; 13.4 g total fat; 99 mg cholesterol; 161 mg sodium. 6.6 g carbohydrates; 28.2 g protein;

# DESSERT

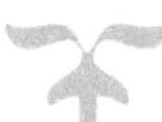

# KETO AVOCADO DESSERT

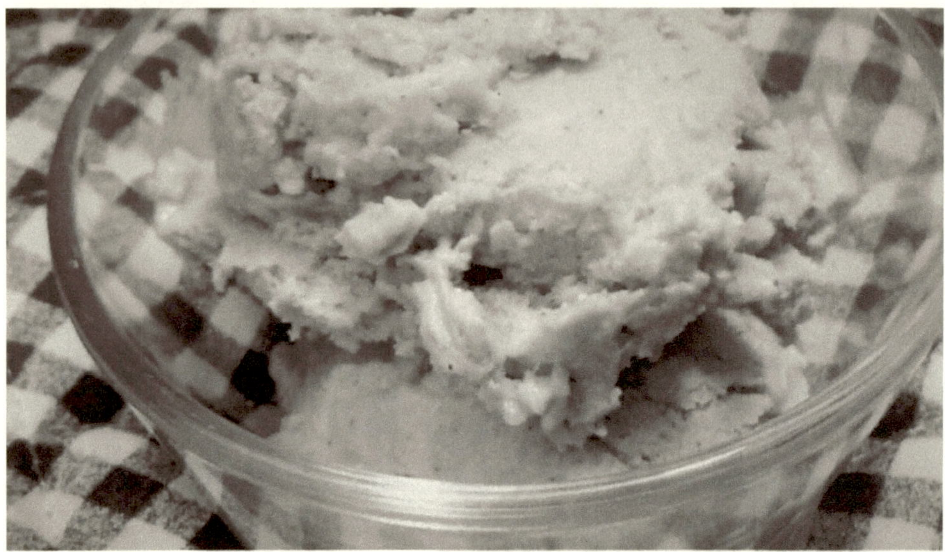

This is a SUPER EASY keto avocado dessert. It's not only easy to make but there's only few ingredients! Low carb, ketogenic and gluten free.

## INGREDIENTS

- 1 ripe avocado - peeled, pitted, and diced
- 1/4 cup heavy whipping cream
- 1/2 teaspoon liquid stevia
- 1/4 teaspoon vanilla extract
- 1/4 teaspoon ground cinnamon

## DIRECTIONS

Prep
10 m

Ready In
1 h 10 m

Servings
2

- Mash avocado in a bowl. Add heavy cream, stevia, vanilla, and cinnamon; mix thoroughly.
- Refrigerate avocado mixture for 1 hour before serving.

## NUTRITION FACTS

Per Serving: 266 calories; 25.7 g fat; 9.7 g carbohydrates; 2.6 g protein; 41 mg cholesterol; 18 mg sodium.

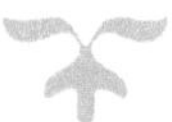

## KETO CHOCOLATE MOUSSE

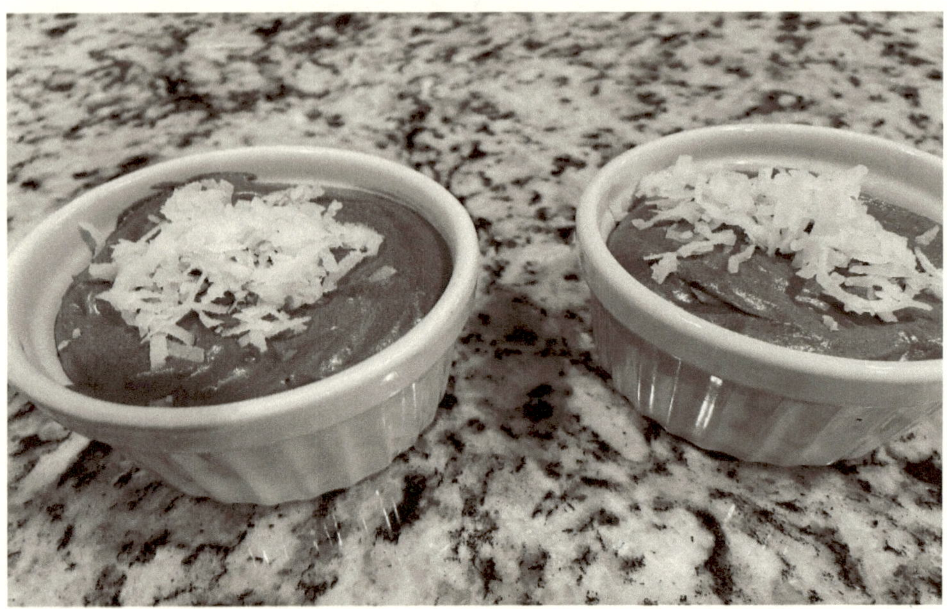

When a sweet craving hits, you'll have this chocolate mousse ready in no time. No need to pre-whip the heavy cream - just throw everything into a bowl and mix! Use any keto-friendly granular sweetener that measures like sugar.

## INGREDIENTS

- 3 ounces cream cheese, softened
- ½ cup heavy cream
- 1 teaspoon vanilla extract

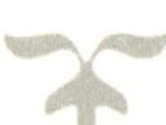

- ¼ cup powdered zero-calorie sweetener (such as Swerve®)
- 2 tablespoons cocoa powder
- 1 pinch salt

# DIRECTIONS

Prep
10 m

Ready In
10 m

Servings
4

- Place cream cheese in a large bowl and beat using an electric mixer until light and fluffy. Turn mixer to low speed and slowly add heavy cream and vanilla extract. Add sweetener, cocoa powder and salt, mixing until well incorporated. Turn mixer to high, and mix until light and fluffy, 1 to 2 minutes more. Serve immediately, or refrigerate for later.

# NUTRITION FACTS

Per Serving: 373 calories; 37.6 g total fat; 128 mg cholesterol; 227 mg sodium. 6.9 g carbohydrates; 5.4 g protein;

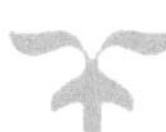

# 90-SECOND KETO BREAD IN A MUG

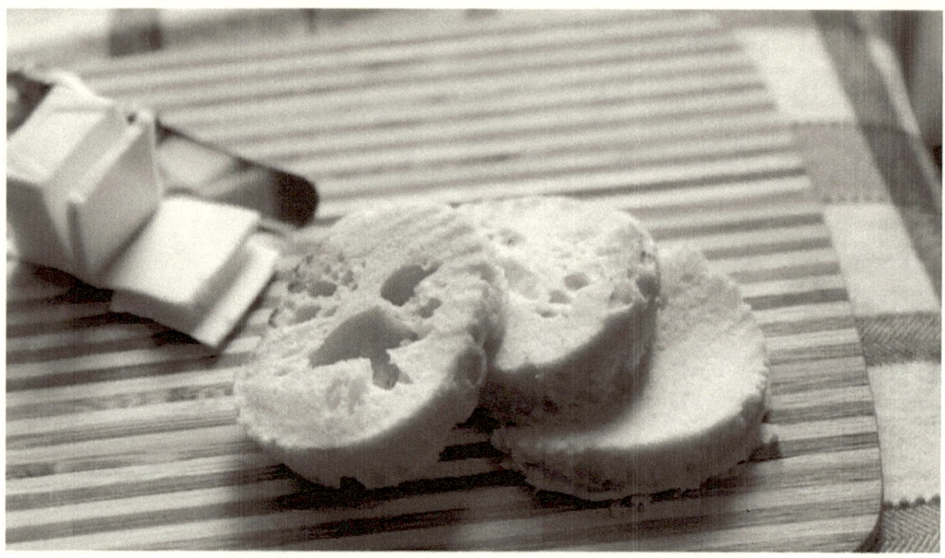

"Try this quick and easy keto and paleo bread made with only 5 ingredients in the microwave in just 90 seconds! So tasty and just perfect for sandwiches and toast."

## INGREDIENTS

- 1 tablespoon butter
- 1/3 cup blanched almond flour
- 1 egg
- 1/2 teaspoon baking powder
- 1 pinch salt

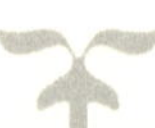

# DIRECTIONS

Prep
5 m

Cook
2 m

Ready In
9 m

Servings
1

- Place butter in a microwave-safe mug. Microwave until melted, about 15 seconds. Swirl mug until fully coated.
- Combine almond flour, egg, baking powder, and salt in the mug; whisk until smooth.
- Microwave at maximum power until set, about 90 seconds. Let cool for 2 minutes before slicing.

# NUTRITION FACTS

Per Serving: 408 calories; 36.4 g fat; 9.8 g carbohydrates; 14.5 g protein; 194 mg cholesterol; 542 mg sodium.

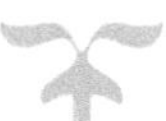

# CAULIFLOWER KETO CASSEROLE

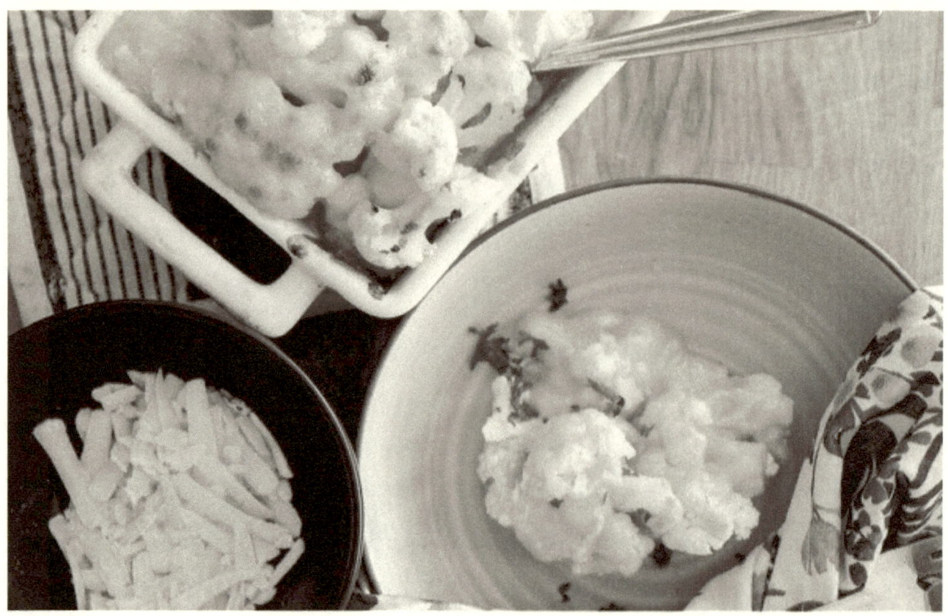

Cauliflower in a creamy cheese sauce is a perfect keto recipe and delicious to boot! Make sure you season well with salt and pepper (nutmeg tastes great as well) otherwise it will taste too bland.

## INGREDIENTS

- ½ head cauliflower florets
- 1 cup shredded Cheddar cheese
- ½ cup heavy cream
- 1 pinch salt and freshly ground black pepper to taste

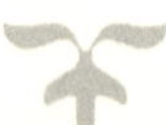

# DIRECTIONS

Prep
10 m

Cook
35 m

Ready In
45 m

Servings
2

- Preheat the oven to 400 degrees F (200 degrees C).

- Bring a large pot of slightly salted water to a boil and cook cauliflower until tender but firm to the bite, about 10 minutes. Drain.

- Combine Cheddar cheese, cream, salt, and pepper in a large bowl. Arrange cauliflower in a casserole dish and cover with cheese mixture.

- Bake in the preheated oven until cheese is bubbly and golden brown, about 25 minutes.

# NUTRITION FACTS

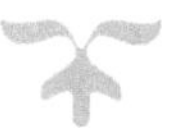

Per Serving: 469 calories; 40.9 g total fat; 141 mg cholesterol; 494 mg sodium. 10 g carbohydrates; 18.1 g protein;

# NO-CHURN KETO ICE CREAM

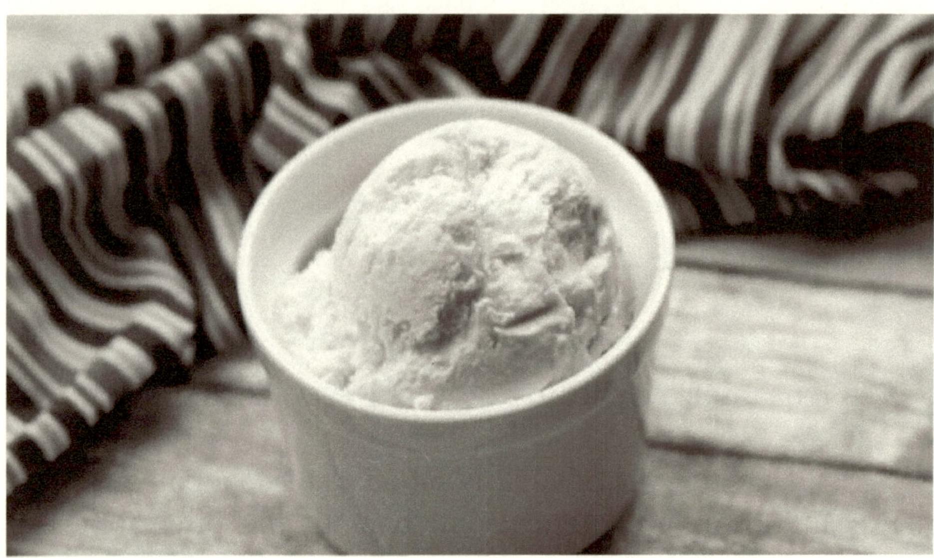

"Quick to make and no ice cream machine needed! After trying different variations of ingredients, I finally figured out a combination that produced a smooth and creamy texture, yet didn't freeze rock-hard like most no-churn ice cream can. The vodka is optional, however it really helps keep the ice cream scoopable and you don't taste it!"

# INGREDIENTS

- 1 cup heavy whipping cream
- 2 tablespoons powdered zero-calorie sweetener
- 1 tablespoon vodka
- 1 teaspoon vanilla extract
- 1/4 teaspoon xanthan gum
- 1 pinch salt

# DIRECTIONS

Prep
10 m

Ready In
3 h 10 m

Servings
3

- Combine cream, sweetener, vodka, vanilla extract, xanthan gum, and salt in a wide-mouth pint-sized jar. Blend cream mixture with an immersion blender in an up-and-down motion until cream has thickened and soft peaks have formed, 60 to 75 seconds. Cover jar and place in the freezer for 3 to 4 hours, stirring every 30 to 40 minutes.

# NUTRITION FACTS

Per Serving: 291 calories; 29.4 g fat; 3.2 g carbohydrates; 1.6 g protein; 109 mg cholesterol; 92 mg sodium.

## TASTY COLLARD GREENS

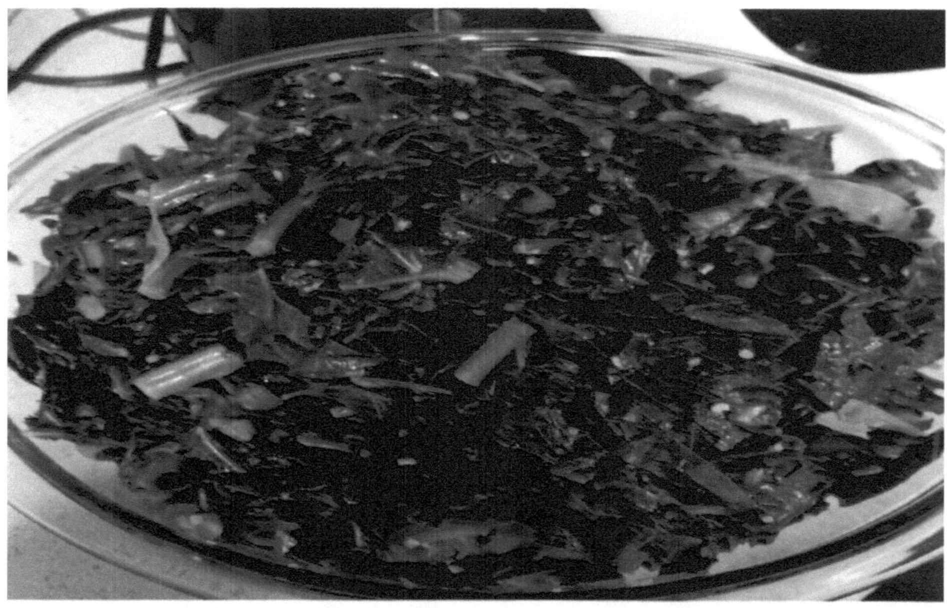

A classic recipe for collard greens that uses smoked turkey to add some flavor. Greens are simmered in chicken stock, then spiced with a dash of red chile flakes.

# INGREDIENTS

- ¼ cup olive oil
- 2 tablespoons minced garlic
- 5 cups chicken stock
- 1 smoked turkey drumstick
- 5 bunches collard greens - rinsed, trimmed and chopped

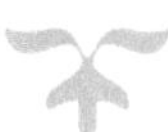

- salt and black pepper to taste
- 1 tablespoon crushed red pepper flakes (optional)

# DIRECTIONS

Prep
30 m

Cook
2 hr

Ready In
2 hr 30 m

Servings
10

- Heat olive oil in a large pot over medium heat. Add garlic, and gently saute until light brown. Pour in the chicken stock, and add the turkey leg. Cover the pot, and simmer for 30 minutes.

- Add the collard greens to the cooking pot, and turn the heat up to medium-high. Let the greens cook down for about 45 minutes, stirring occasionally.

- Reduce heat to medium, and season with salt and pepper to taste. Continue to cook until the greens are tender and dark green, 45 to 60 minutes. Drain greens, reserving liquid. Mix in red pepper flakes if desired. Use liquid to reheat leftovers.

## NUTRITION FACTS

Per Serving: 142 calories; 7.9 g total fat; 23 mg cholesterol; 689 mg sodium. 10.6 g carbohydrates; 9.6 g protein;

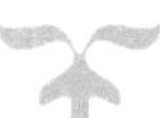

# SAUSAGE STUFFED JALAPENOS

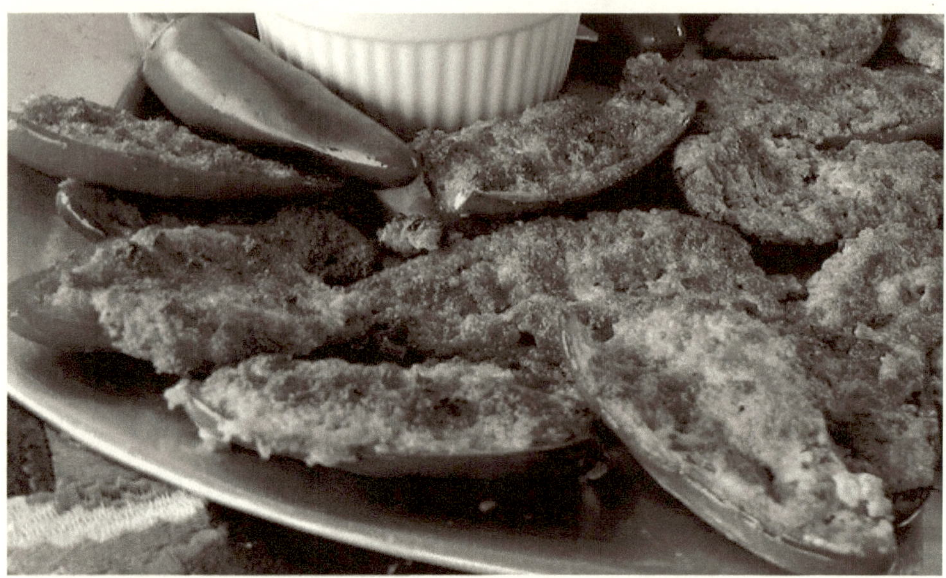

Jalapeno pepper halves are stuffed with cheese and sausage. You will love this spicy appetizer treat!

## INGREDIENTS

- 1 pound ground pork sausage
- 1 (8 ounce) package cream cheese, softened
- 1 cup shredded Parmesan cheese
- 1 pound large fresh jalapeno peppers, halved lengthwise and seeded
- 1 (8 ounce) bottle Ranch dressing (optional)

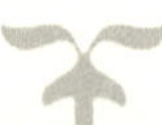

# DIRECTIONS

Prep
25 m

Cook
20 m

Ready In
45 m

Servings
12

- Preheat oven to 425 degrees F (220 degrees C).

- Place sausage in a skillet over medium heat, and cook until evenly brown. Drain grease.

- In a bowl, mix the sausage, cream cheese, and Parmesan cheese. Spoon about 1 tablespoon sausage mixture into each jalapeno half. Arrange stuffed halves in baking dishes.

- Bake 20 minutes in the preheated oven, until bubbly and lightly browned. Serve with Ranch dressing.

# NUTRITION FACTS

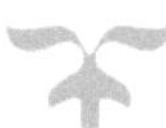

Per Serving: 362 calories; 34.3 g total fat; 58 mg cholesterol; 601 mg sodium. 4.3 g carbohydrates; 9.2 g protein;

# GRILLED ASPARAGUS

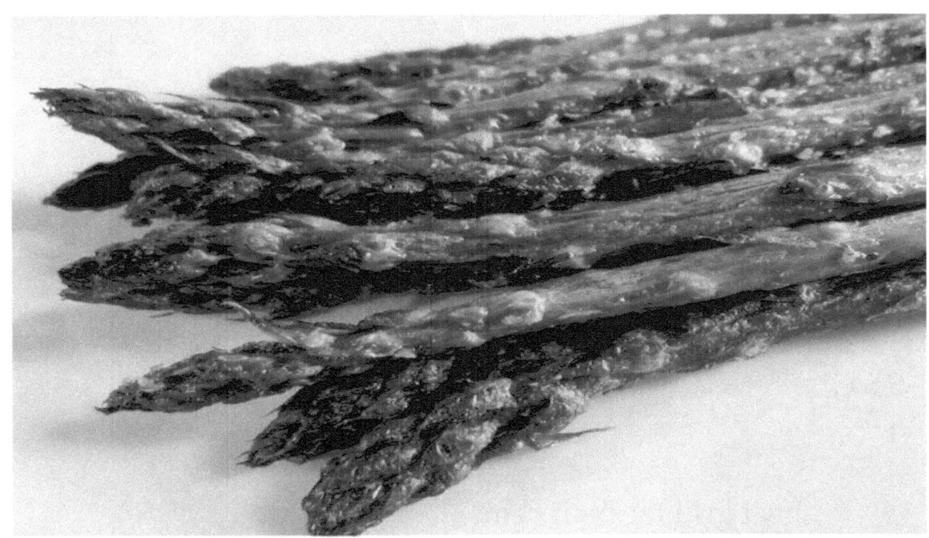

The special thing about this recipe is that it's so simple. Fresh asparagus with a little oil, salt, and pepper is cooked quickly over high heat on the grill. Enjoy the natural flavor of your veggies.

## INGREDIENTS

- 1 pound fresh asparagus spears, trimmed
- 1 tablespoon olive oil
- salt and pepper to taste

# DIRECTIONS

Prep
15 m

Cook
3 m

Ready In
18 m

Servings
4

- Preheat grill for high heat.

- Lightly coat the asparagus spears with olive oil. Season with salt and pepper to taste.

- Grill over high heat for 2 to 3 minutes, or to desired tenderness.

# NUTRITION FACTS

Per Serving: 53 calories; 3.5 g total fat; 0 mg cholesterol; 2 mg sodium. 4.4 g carbohydrates; 2.5 g protein;

# PRETZEL TURTLES

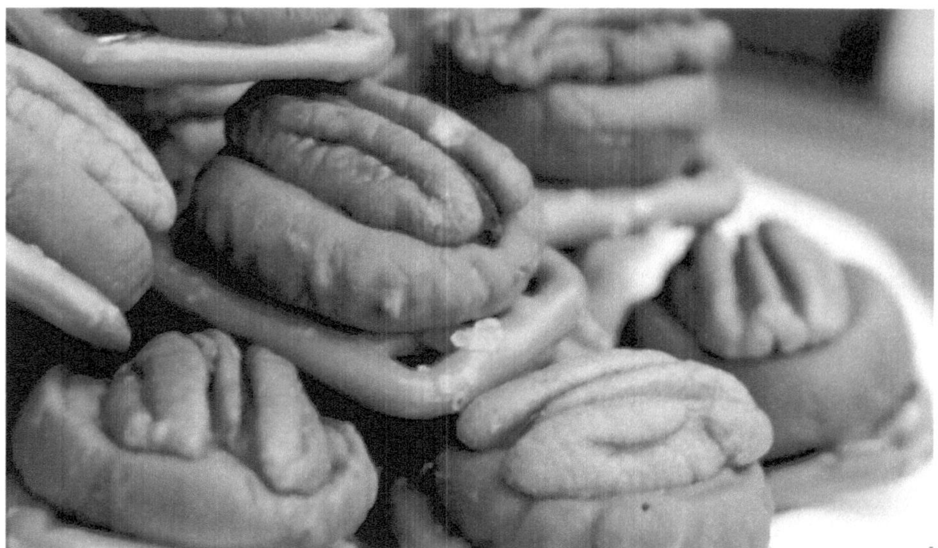

"Quick and easy Turtles® candies! Mini pretzels, caramel covered chocolate candies, and pecans make up this delicious treat."

## INGREDIENTS

- 20 small mini pretzels
- 20 chocolate covered caramel candies
- 20 pecan halves

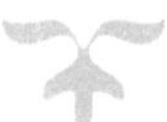

# DIRECTIONS

Prep
10 m

Cook
4 m

Ready In
14 m

Servings
20

- Preheat oven to 300 degrees F (150 degrees C).
- Arrange the pretzels in a single layer on a parchment lined cookie sheet. Place one chocolate covered caramel candy on each pretzel.
- Bake for 4 minutes. While the candy is warm, press a pecan half onto each candy covered pretzel. Cool completely before storing in an airtight container.

## NUTRITION FACTS

Per Serving: 82 calories; 2.2 g fat; 14.1 g carbohydrates; 1.7 g protein; < 1 mg cholesterol; 263 mg sodium.

# PUMPKIN PIE SPICE I

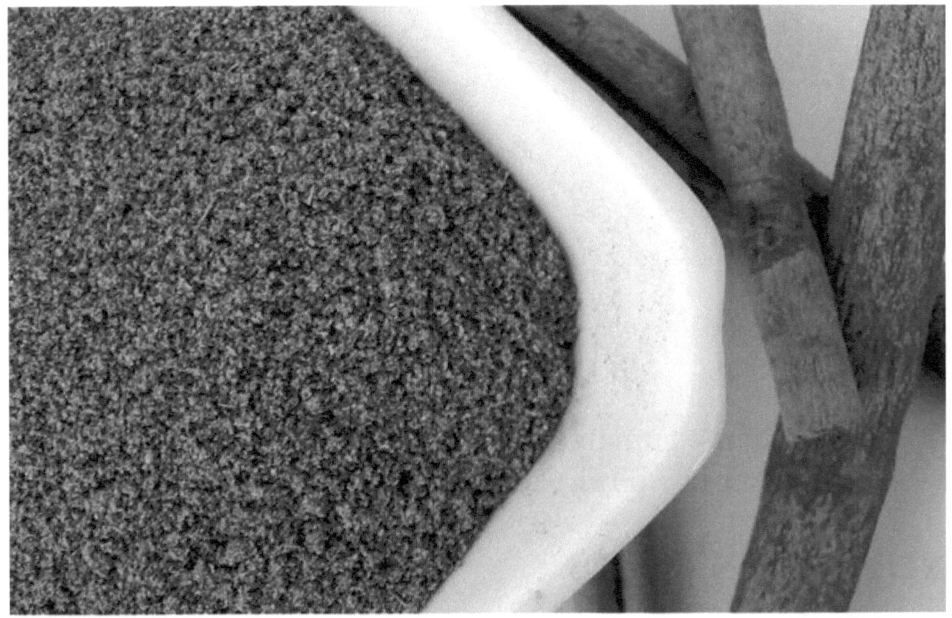

Use this mixture in recipes that call for pumpkin pie spice. A blend of cinnamon, nutmeg, ginger and allspice that can be scaled to any size.

## INGREDIENTS

- ¼ cup ground cinnamon
- 4 teaspoons ground nutmeg
- 4 teaspoons ground ginger
- 1 tablespoon ground allspice

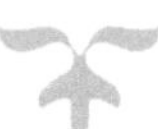

# DIRECTIONS

Prep
1 m

Ready In
1 m

Servings
8

- Combine cinnamon, nutmeg, ginger, and allspice together in a bowl. Store in air-tight container.

# NUTRITION FACTS

Per Serving: 21 calories; 0.7 g total fat; 0 mg cholesterol; 1 mg sodium. 4.7 g carbohydrates; 0.4 g protein;

# HOMESTYLE TURKEY, THE MICHIGANDER WAY

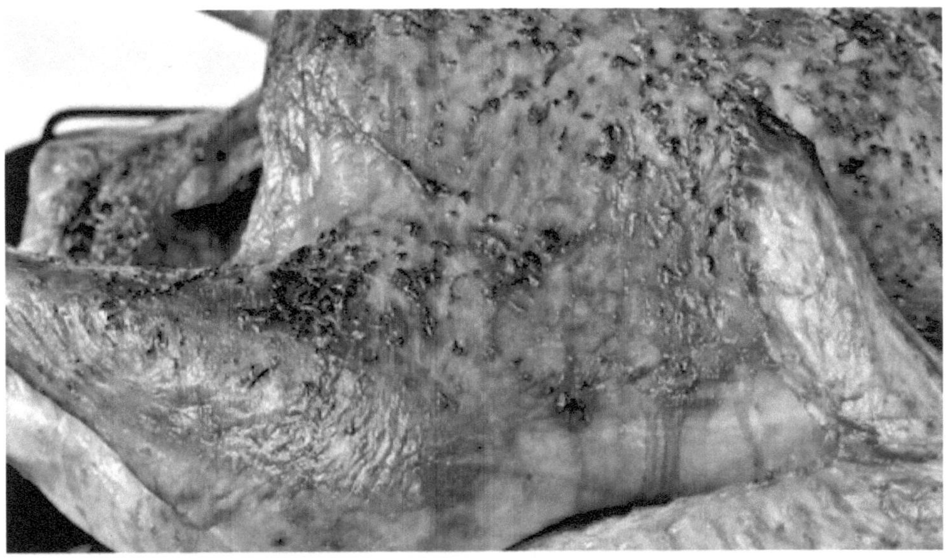

"A simple, down to basics recipe when it comes to the good old tom turkey."

## INGREDIENTS

- 1 (12 pound) whole turkey
- 6 tablespoons butter, divided
- 4 cups warm water
- 3 tablespoons chicken bouillon
- 2 tablespoons dried parsley

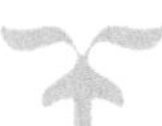

- 2 tablespoons dried minced onion
- 2 tablespoons seasoning salt

# DIRECTIONS

Prep
10 m

Cook
5 h

Ready In
5 h 10 m

Servings
16

- Preheat oven to 350 degrees F (175 degrees C). Rinse and wash turkey. Discard the giblets, or add to pan if they are anyone's favorites.
- Place turkey in a Dutch oven or roasting pan. Separate the skin over the breast to make little pockets. Put 3 tablespoons of the butter on both sides between the skin and breast meat. This makes for very juicy breast meat.
- In a medium bowl, combine the water with the bouillon. Sprinkle in the parsley and minced onion. Pour over the top of the turkey. Sprinkle seasoning salt over the turkey.

- Cover with foil, and bake in the preheated oven 3 1/2 to 4 hours, until the internal temperature of the turkey reaches 180 degrees F (80 degrees C). For the last 45 minutes or so, remove the foil so the turkey will brown nicely.

## NUTRITION FACTS

Per Serving: 545 calories; 27.9 g fat; 0.9 g carbohydrates; 68.1 g protein; 210 mg cholesterol; 560 mg sodium.

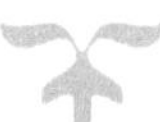

# FABULOUS BEEF TENDERLOIN

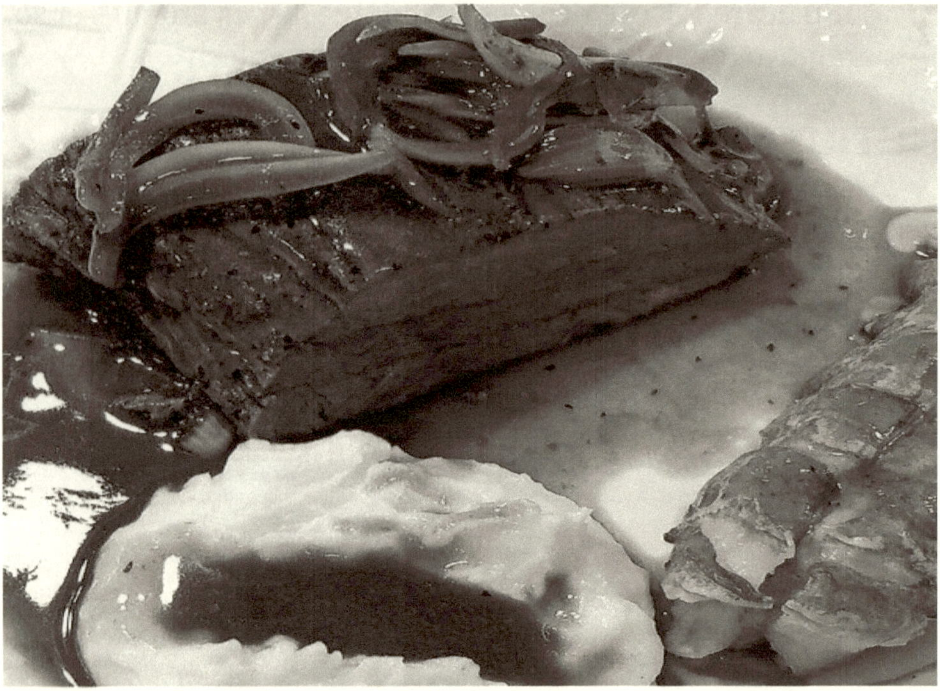

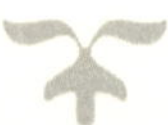

This beef tenderloin will melt in your mouth. We've had it for both of our Christmas dinners this year (2 families) and got RAVE reviews from everyone. Hard to believe it's so easy to prepare!

## INGREDIENTS

- 1 (3 pound) beef tenderloin roast
- ¾ cup soy sauce

- ½ cup melted butter

## DIRECTIONS

Prep
5 m

Cook
45 m

Ready In
1 h

Servings
6

- Preheat oven to 350 degrees F (175 degrees C).

- Place roast into a shallow, glass baking dish. Pour soy sauce and melted butter over the tenderloin.

- Bake in preheated oven for 10 minutes, then turn the roast over, and continue cooking 35 to 40 minutes, basting occasionally until the internal temperature of the roast is at 140 degrees F (60 degrees C) for medium. Or, cook to your desired degree of doneness. Let meat rest for 10 to 15 minutes before slicing.

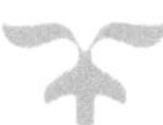

# NUTRITION FACTS

Per Serving: 591 calories; 33.2 g total fat; 220 mg cholesterol; 2047 mg sodium. 2.4 g carbohydrates; 66.9 g protein;

## ROASTED GARLIC CAULIFLOWER

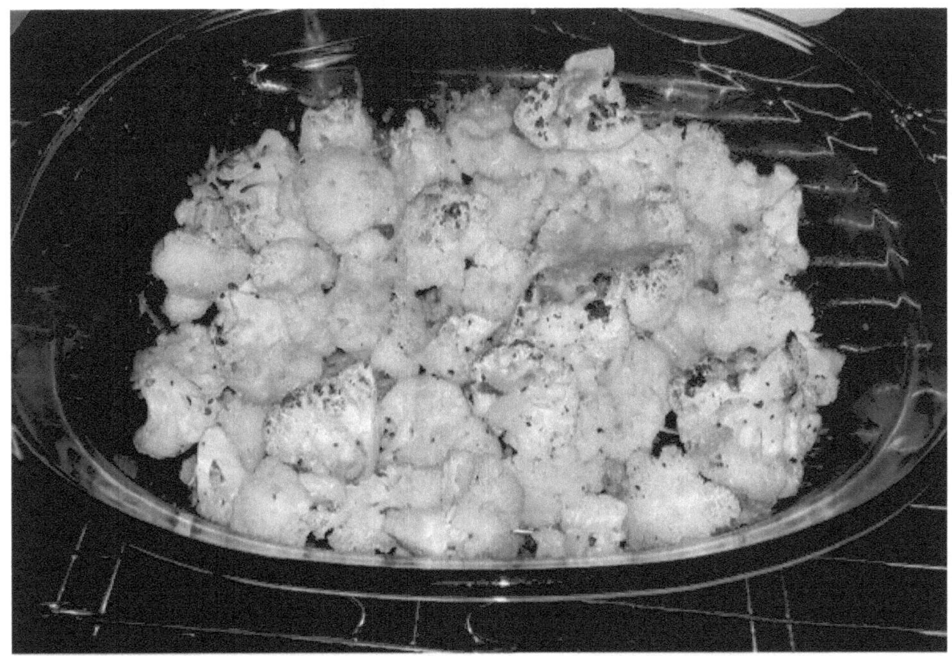

Roasted garlic cauliflower is the best roasted cauliflower recipe ever! Super easy with 5 minute prep. You'll love this simple, improved method for how to roast cauliflower in the oven.

# INGREDIENTS

- 2 tablespoons minced garlic
- 3 tablespoons olive oil
- 1 large head cauliflower, separated into florets
- ⅓ cup grated Parmesan cheese

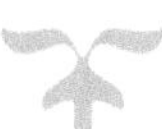

- salt and black pepper to taste
- 1 tablespoon chopped fresh parsley

# DIRECTIONS

Prep
15 m

Cook
25 m

Ready In
40 m

Servings
6

- Preheat the oven to 450 degrees F (220 degrees C). Grease a large casserole dish.

- Place the olive oil and garlic in a large resealable bag. Add cauliflower, and shake to mix. Pour into the prepared casserole dish, and season with salt and pepper to taste.

- Bake for 25 minutes, stirring halfway through. Top with Parmesan cheese and parsley, and broil for 3 to 5 minutes, until golden brown.

# NUTRITION FACTS

Per Serving: 118 calories; 8.2 g total fat; 4 mg cholesterol; 111 mg sodium. 8.6 g carbohydrates; 4.7 g protein;

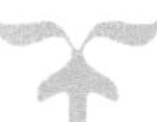

# PINA COLADA COOKIES I

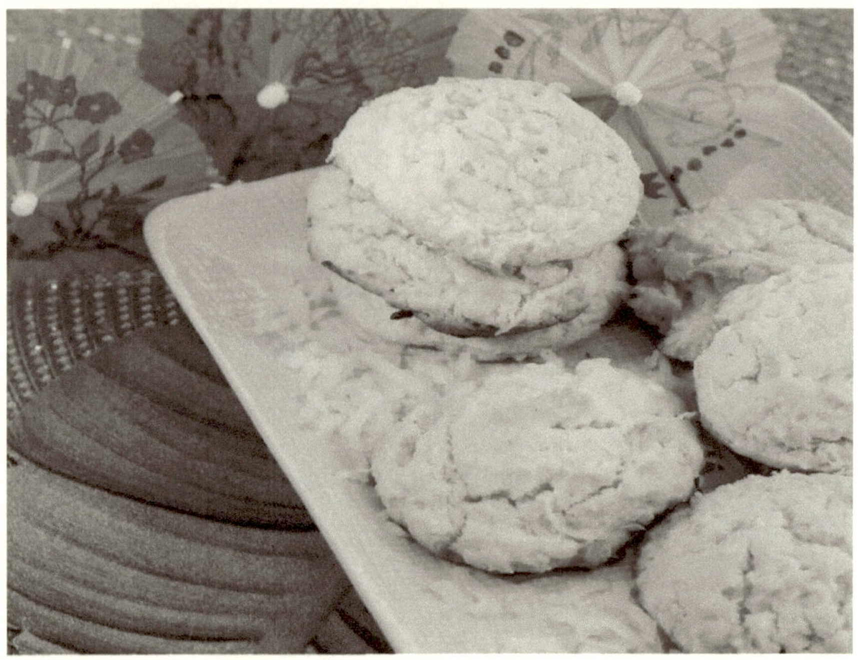

A pineapple-coconut cookie with a hint of rum. I started out to make a plain pineapple cookie but then got daring and in the process I discovered a great cookie.

## INGREDIENTS

- 1 tablespoon and 1 teaspoon minced garlic
- 2 tablespoons olive oil
- 5/8 large head cauliflower, separated into florets

- 2 tablespoons and 2-1/2 teaspoons grated Parmesan cheese
- salt and black pepper to taste
- 2 teaspoons chopped fresh parsley

# DIRECTIONS

Servings
4

- Preheat oven to 350 degrees F (175 degrees C).

- Cut the softened margarine or butter into the cake mix. Use a fork mash them together until they are well combined and the mixture resembles coarse crumbs. Beat in the eggs, milk and rum extract and mix well. Stir in the flaked coconut until combined.

- Drop by teaspoonfuls onto an ungreased baking sheet and bake at 350 degrees F (175 degrees C) for 12 to 15 minutes.

## NUTRITION FACTS

Per Serving: 70 calories; 3.3 g total fat; 13 mg cholesterol; 88 mg sodium. 9.5 g carbohydrates; 0.6 g protein;

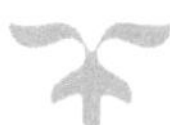

# PUMPKIN SPICE

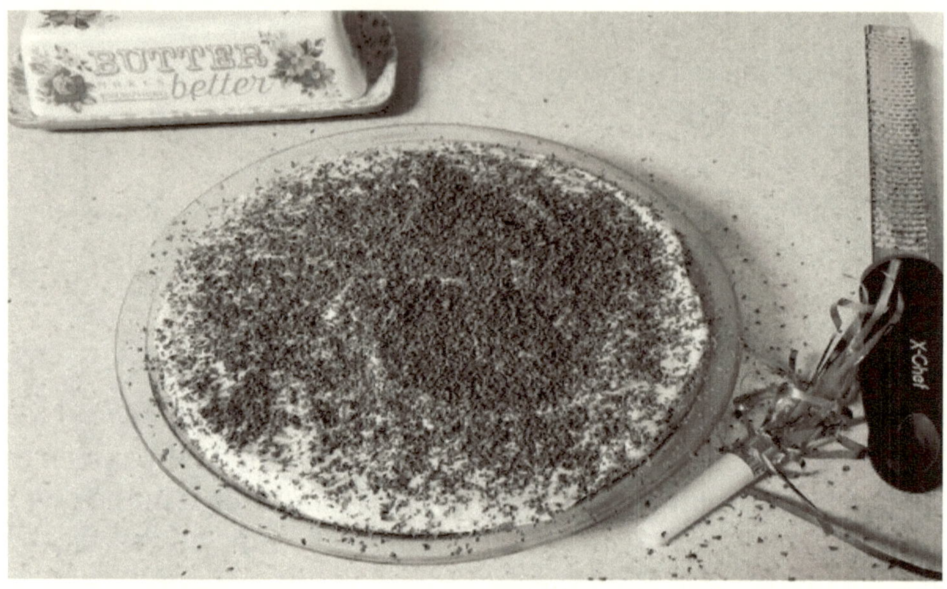

This will make enough for one recipe of pumpkin pie. But you could increase amounts to keep a mix on hand. These spices added to a pumpkin pie make the dish as far as I am concerned.

## INGREDIENTS

- 1 teaspoon ground cinnamon
- ¼ teaspoon ground nutmeg
- ¼ teaspoon ground ginger
- ⅛ teaspoon ground cloves

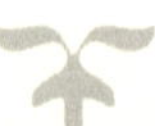

# DIRECTIONS

Prep
2 m

Ready In
2 m

Servings
2

- In a small bowl, mix together cinnamon, nutmeg, ginger and cloves. Store in an airtight container.

# NUTRITION FACTS

Per Serving: 6 calories; 0.2 g total fat; 0 mg cholesterol; 1 mg sodium. 1.4 g carbohydrates; 0.1 g protein;

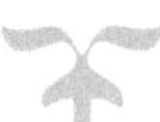

# RAW CANDY

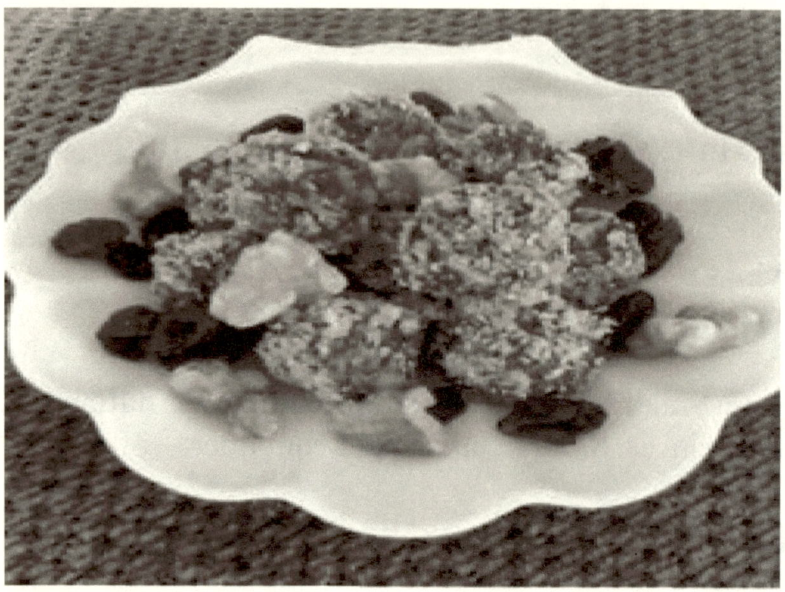

This will make enough for one recipe of pumpkin pie. "Sweet treats with no added sugar! Unfired fare that is all natural and vegan!"

## INGREDIENTS

- 1 cup raisins
- 1 cup walnuts
- 1 tablespoon vegetable oil
- 1 cup sliced almonds

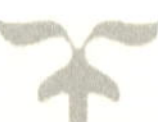

# DIRECTIONS

Prep
20 m

Ready In
20 m

Servings
4

- In a food processor combine raisins and walnuts. Process until they form a sticky ball.
- Coat hands with oil and roll mixture into balls the size of large marbles, then coat with sliced almonds.
- Cover and refrigerate for up to 3 days.

## NUTRITION FACTS

Per Serving: 45 calories; 3.5 g fat; 3.2 g carbohydrates; 1 g protein; 0 mg cholesterol; < 1 mg sodium.

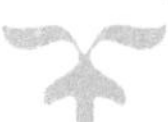

# PUMPKIN COOKIE DIP

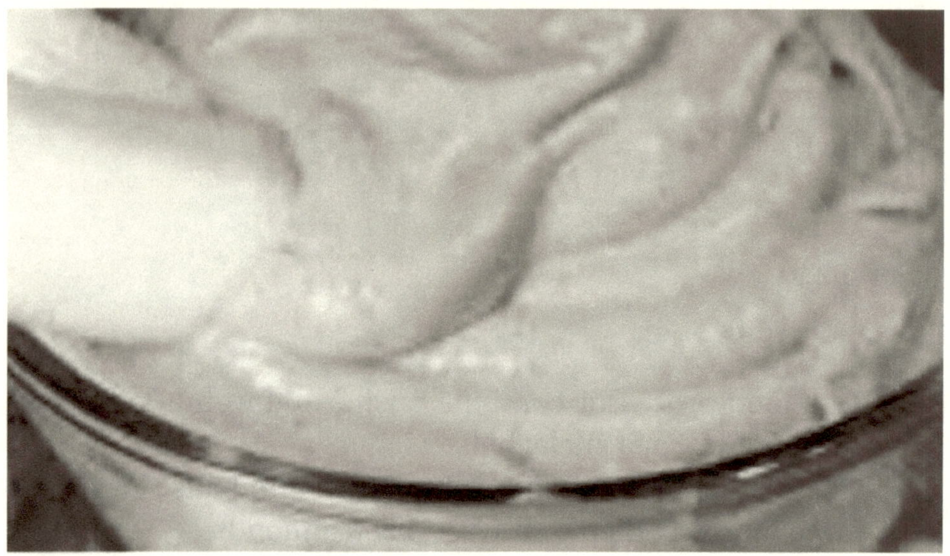

A few moments are all you need to whip up this creamy pumpkin dip that goes perfectly with gingersnap cookies.

## INGREDIENTS

- 1 (8 ounce) package cream cheese, softened
- 2 (7 ounce) jars marshmallow creme
- 1 (15 ounce) can solid pack pumpkin
- 1 teaspoon ground cinnamon

# DIRECTIONS

Prep
10 m

Ready In
10 m

Servings
4

- In a medium bowl, beat together cream cheese and marshmallow creme until smooth. Fold in pumpkin and cinnamon. Cover, and chill in the refrigerator until serving.

# NUTRITION FACTS

Per Serving: 46 calories; 1.7 g fat; 7.3 g carbohydrates; 0.5 g protein; 5 mg cholesterol; 42 mg sodium.

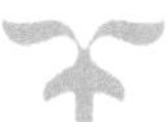

## POPCORN MACAROONS

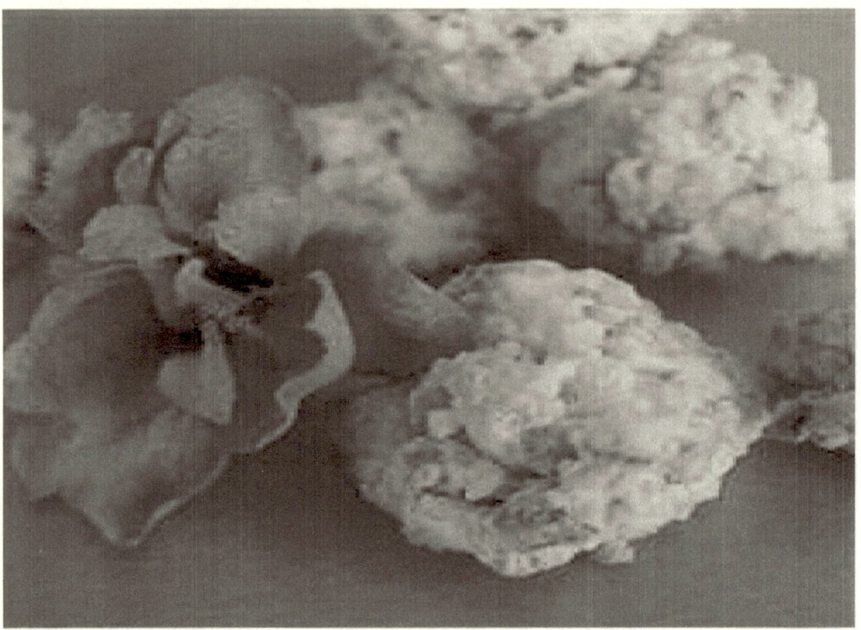

This is a wonderful macaroon recipe! We recommend a sugar substitute that is heat stable using a sweetener such as sucralose or acesulfame potassium.

## INGREDIENTS

- 3 tablespoons and 1-3/4 teaspoons popped popcorn
- 3/8 egg whites
- 1/8 teaspoon baking powder
- 1/8 teaspoon salt

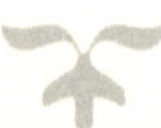

- 1/8 teaspoon cream of tartar
- 3/4 teaspoon granulated artificial sweetener

# DIRECTIONS

Prep
10 m

Cook
12 m

Ready In
25 m

Servings
4

- Preheat oven to 350 degrees F (175 degrees C). Lightly grease cookie sheets. Place popped popcorn into a food processor or blender; grind into small kernels.

- In a large bowl, whip egg whites until frothy. Add baking powder, salt and cream of tartar; continue whipping to stiff peaks. Gradually mix in the sugar substitute. Fold in the popcorn pieces. Drop by teaspoonfuls onto the prepared cookie sheets.

- Bake for 12 to 15 minutes in the preheated oven, or until lightly browned. Allow cookies to cool on cookie sheets before removing.

## NUTRITION FACTS

Per Serving: 8 calories; 0.3 g total fat; 0 mg cholesterol; 32 mg sodium. 0.3 g carbohydrates; 1.1 g protein;

# MINI MERINGUES

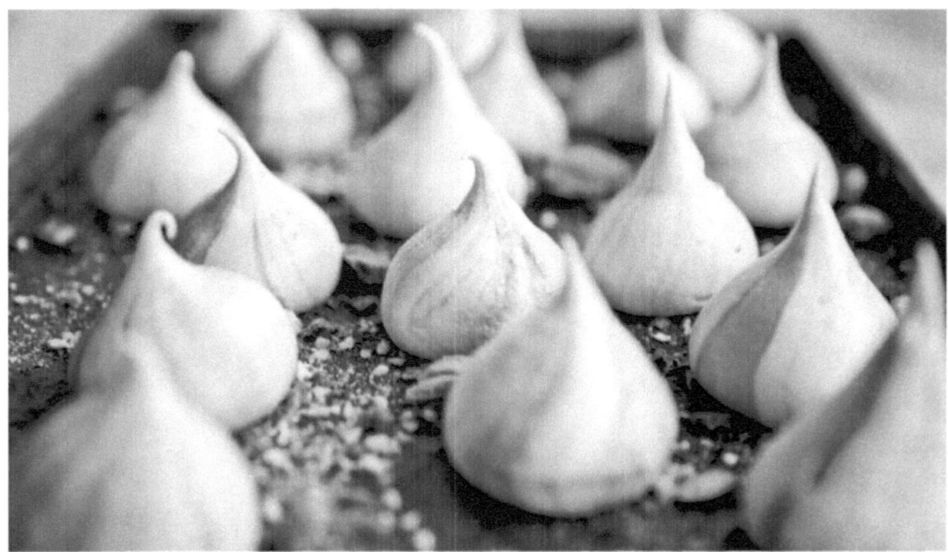

These crunchy dainties are great with coffee or with cream for dessert. And they're low fat! Substitute 2 teaspoons instant coffee granules or 1 1/2 tablespoons cocoa for the vanilla if you like. Coffee kisses are great sandwiched together with melted white or dark chocolate. Spooned vanilla ones are good with cream and chocolate ones are good as finger biscuits with coffee.

## INGREDIENTS

- 5/8 egg whites
- 2 tablespoons and 2 teaspoons superfine sugar
- 1/4 teaspoon vanilla extract

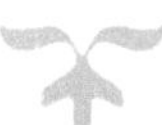

# DIRECTIONS

Prep
20 m

Cook
40 m

Ready In
1 hr

Servings
4

- Preheat oven to 300 degrees F (150 degrees C). Line a baking sheet with parchment paper.

- In large bowl, beat egg whites until stiff, but not dry. Gradually beat in sugar until a little of the mixture between your thumb and forefinger feels smooth, not gritty. Stir in vanilla. Pipe or spoon small portions onto baking tray and bake 35 minutes, or until dry but not brown. Turn off oven and leave meringues to cool inside.

# NUTRITION FACTS

Per Serving: 36 calories; 0 g total fat; 0 mg cholesterol; 9 mg sodium. 8.4 g carbohydrates; 0.6 g protein;

# GET WELL CUSTARD

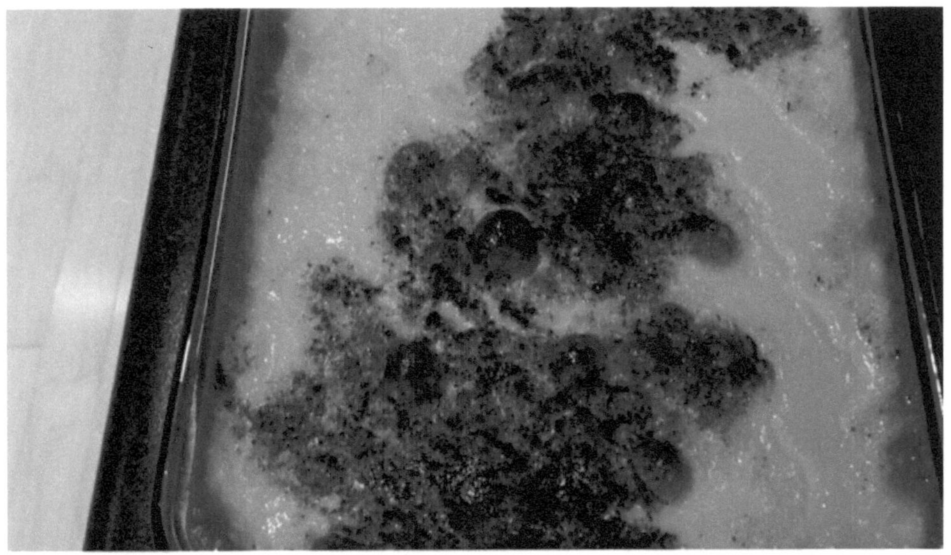

"This simple custard is wonderful when you are not feeling well, but adapted with half-and-half and no-carb sweetener, it makes a great change on a low-carb diet."

## INGREDIENTS

- 4 eggs
- 1/2 cup white sugar
- 1/4 teaspoon salt
- 1 teaspoon vanilla extract
- 4 cups warm milk
- ground nutmeg

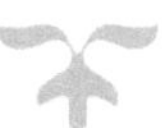

# DIRECTIONS

Prep
15 m

Cook
55 m

Ready In
1 h 10 m

Servings
4

- Preheat oven to 350 degrees F (175 degrees C).
- Beat eggs with sugar, salt, and vanilla in a bowl. Slowly whisk warm milk into the egg mixture. Pour through a strainer into a 1 1/2-quart round baking dish. Sprinkle nutmeg over the mixture. Place the baking dish into a larger pan. Pour about 1 inch of water into the larger pan.
- Bake in the preheated oven until a knife inserted into the center comes out clean, 55 to 60 minutes. Cool to room temperature. Chill to serve.

# NUTRITION FACTS

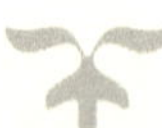

Per Serving: 118 calories; 3.9 g fat; 14.8 g carbohydrates; 5.7 g protein; 82 mg cholesterol; 126 mg sodium.

# KETO PEANUT BUTTER COOKIES

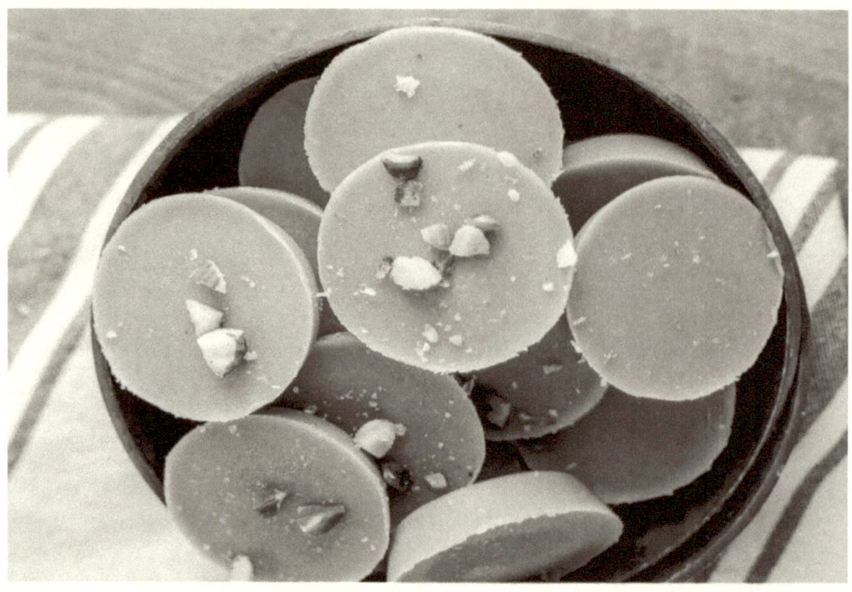

This is a great keto dessert with only 3 ingredients. If you want you can sweeten it with stevia or other sweeteners, but the peanut butter is sweet enough.

## INGREDIENTS

- 1/3 cup and 1 tablespoon unsweetened peanut butter, softened
- 1/3 cup and 1 tablespoon coconut oil
- 1 tablespoon and 1-3/4 teaspoons unsweetened vanilla-flavored almond milk

- 3-3/4 cups vanilla liquid stevia, or as needed (optional)

# DIRECTIONS

Prep
10 m

Cook
2 hr

Ready In
2 h 10 m

Servings
4

- Line a loaf pan with parchment paper.

- Combine peanut butter and coconut oil in a microwave-safe dish. Microwave 30 seconds until slightly melted. Add to blender with almond milk and stevia; blend until well combined. Pour into loaf pan and refrigerate until set, about 2 hours.

## NUTRITION FACTS

Per Serving: 341 calories; 34.9 g total fat; 0 mg cholesterol; 122 mg sodium. 5.3 g carbohydrates; 6.5 g protein;

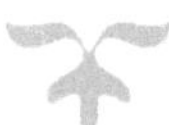

# KETO PEANUT COOKIES

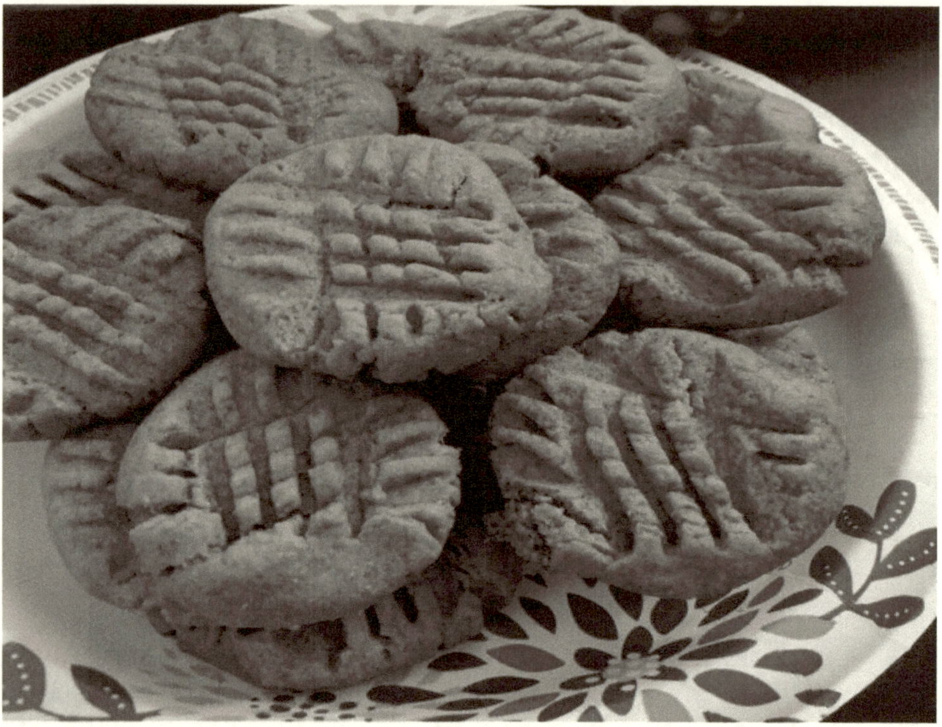

Kids will love these scrumptious low-carb keto cookies; all you need is peanut butter, vanilla extract, an egg, and some sugar substitute.

## INGREDIENTS

- 1/3 cup peanut butter

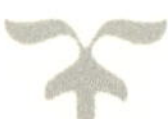

- 38 cups low-calorie natural sweetener (such as Swerve®)
- 3/8 egg
- 1/4 teaspoon sugar-free vanilla extract

# DIRECTIONS

Prep
10 m

Cook
15 m

Ready In
25 m

Servings
4

- Preheat oven to 350 degrees F (175 degrees C). Line a baking sheet with parchment paper.

- Combine peanut butter, sweetener, egg, and vanilla extract in a bowl; mix well until a dough is formed.

- Roll dough into 1-inch balls. Place on the prepared baking sheet and press down twice with a fork in a criss-cross pattern.

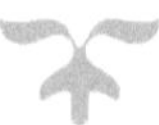

- Bake in the the preheated oven until edges are golden, 12 to 15 minutes. Cool on the baking sheet for 1 minute before removing to a wire rack to cool completely.

## NUTRITION FACTS

Per Serving: 133 calories; 11.2 g total fat; 16 mg cholesterol; 105 mg sodium. 12.4 g carbohydrates; 5.9 g protein;

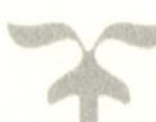

# CREAM PUFF SHELLS

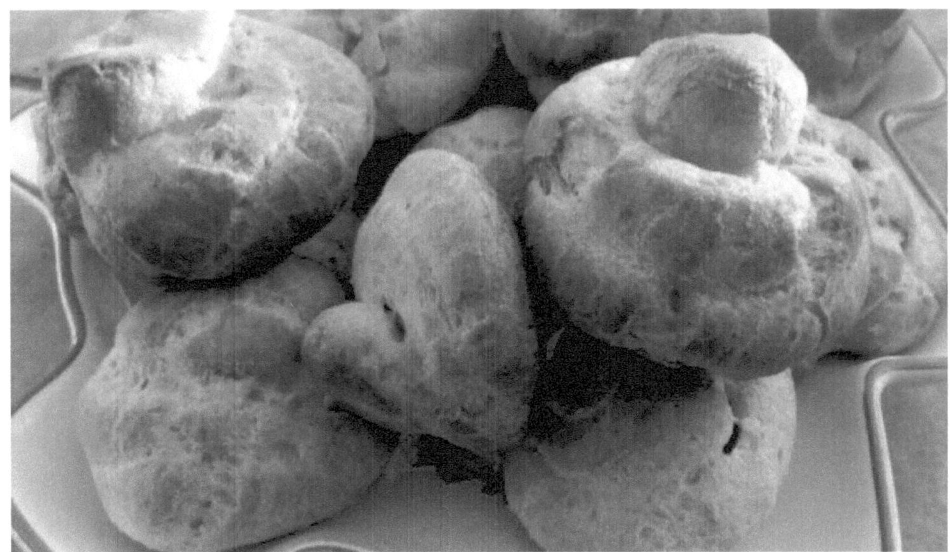

"Choux pastry -- fill with sweetened whipped cream or custard."

## INGREDIENTS

- 1/2 cup shortening
- 1/8 teaspoon salt
- 1 cup boiling water
- 1 cup sifted all-purpose flour
- 4 eggs

# DIRECTIONS

Prep
20 m

Cook
40 m

Ready In
1 h

Servings
12

- Preheat oven to 450 degrees F (230 degrees C). In medium saucepan, combine shortening, salt and boiling water and heat until entire mixture boils. Reduce heat, add flour all at once and stir vigorously until mixture forms a ball. Remove from heat and add eggs, one at a time, beating thoroughly after each addition. Continue beating until mixture is thick and shiny and breaks from spoon.
- Pipe or spoon onto ungreased cookie sheet and bake 20 minutes, reduce heat to 350 degrees F (175 degrees C) and bake 20 minutes more, or until golden and sound hollow when tapped. Cool and fill.

# NUTRITION FACTS

Per Serving: 137 calories; 10.3 g fat; 8.1 g carbohydrates; 3.2 g protein; 62 mg cholesterol; 48 mg sodium.

# CREAM CHEESE TART SHELLS

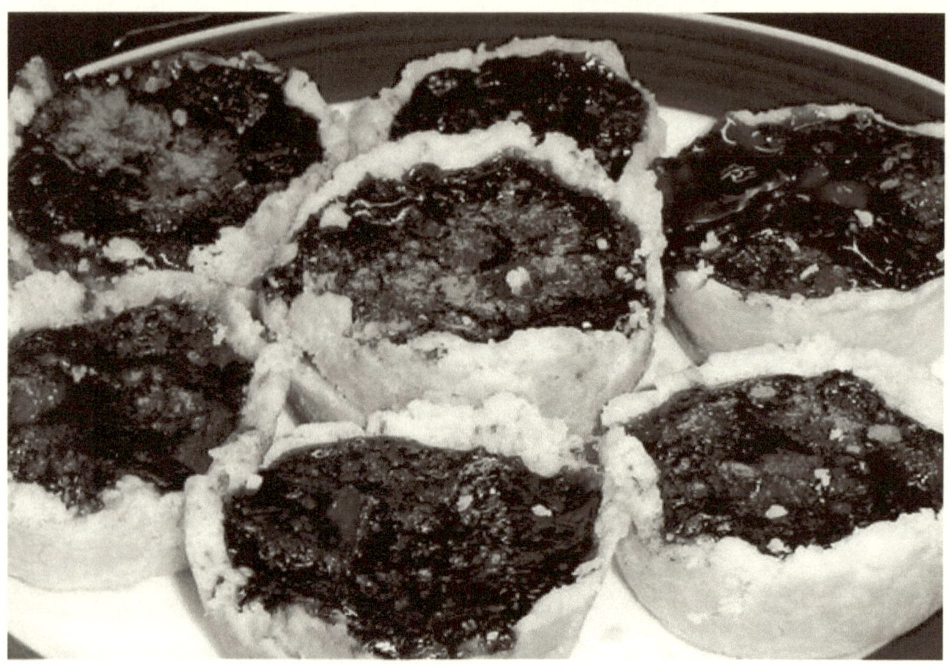

Cream cheese adds a deliciously rich flavor to these tart shells.

## INGREDIENTS

- 1/2 ounce cream cheese, softened
- 1 tablespoon and 1 teaspoon butter, softened
- 2 tablespoons and 2 teaspoons all-purpose flour

# DIRECTIONS

Prep
40 m

Cook
20 m

Ready In
2 hr

Servings
4

- Blend cream cheese and butter or margarine. Stir in flour just until blended. Chill about 1 hour. This can be made ahead and chilled for up to 24 hours.
- Preheat oven to 325 degrees F (165 degrees C).
- Shape dough into 24 one-inch balls and press into ungreased 1 1/2 inch muffin cups (mini-muffin size) to make a shallow shell. Fill with your favorite filling and bake for 20 minutes, or until the crust is light brown.

# NUTRITION FACTS

Per Serving: 65 calories; 5.1 g total fat; 14 mg cholesterol; 38 mg sodium. 4.1 g carbohydrates; 0.8 g protein;

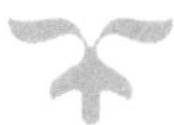

# LOW CARB FLAVORED MERINGUE COOKIES

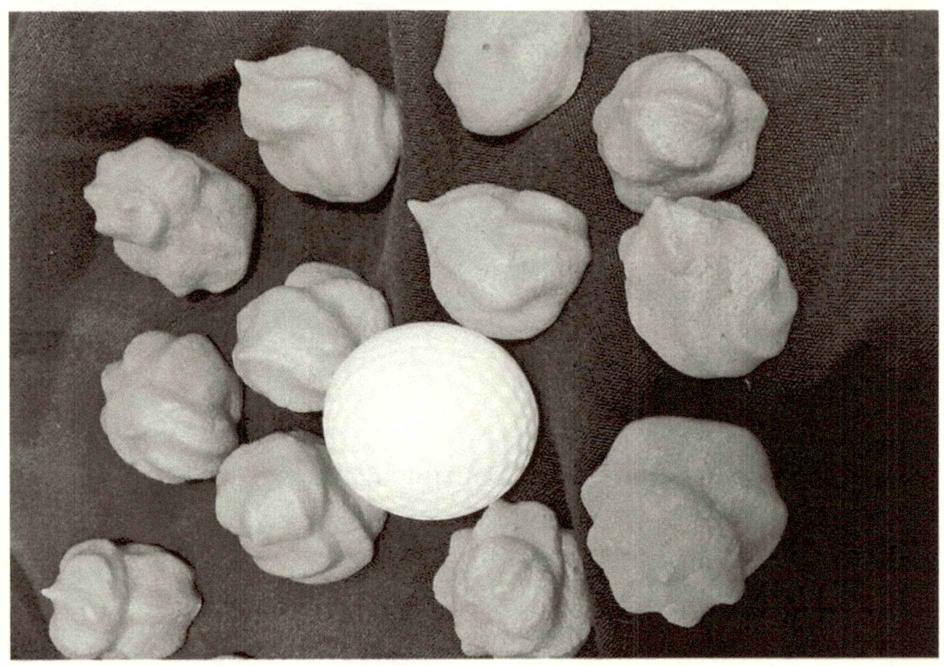

Cream cheese adds a deliciously rich flavor to these tart shells.

## INGREDIENTS

- 1/2 cup and 2 teaspoons sugar-free strawberry Jell-O® mix

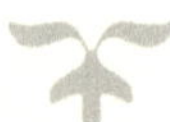

- 2 tablespoons and 2 teaspoons granulated no-calorie sugar substitute
- 1 egg whites at room temperature
- 1/8 teaspoon cream of tartar
- 1/8 teaspoon salt

## DIRECTIONS

Prep
10 m

Cook
1 hr 30 m

Ready In
2 hr 15 m

Servings
4

- Preheat oven to 250 degrees F (120 degrees C). Line 2 baking sheets with parchment paper.
- Cut about 1/4 inch off a corner of a heavy gallon-size resealable plastic bag, and push a large-size cake decorating tip (such as a star tip) into the opening. The fit should be tight.
- In a small bowl, stir the gelatin mix with the sugar substitute. In a large bowl, using an electric mixer, beat the

egg whites with cream of tartar and salt until stiff peaks form. As you beat the egg whites, gradually add the gelatin mixture, about 1 tablespoon at a time. Spoon the fluffy mixture into the prepared plastic bag, and gently squeeze and twist the bag to force the meringue mixture to the decorating tip. (Do not seal bag, so that air can escape.)

- Squeeze the bag to place golf-ball size dollops of meringue mixture onto the prepared baking sheets. For a decorative effect, twist and lift as you place the cookie on the sheet, to make a pretty shape.
- Bake in the preheated oven until the cookies are set and dry, about 1 hour and 30 minutes. Do not open oven door while baking. At end of baking time, turn off oven, open oven door, and allow the cookies to slowly cool in the oven before removing from baking sheets. Store in airtight container.

## NUTRITION FACTS

Per Serving: 5 calories; 0 g total fat; 0 mg cholesterol; 41 mg sodium. 0.1 g carbohydrates; 1 g protein;

# PUDDING COOKIES I

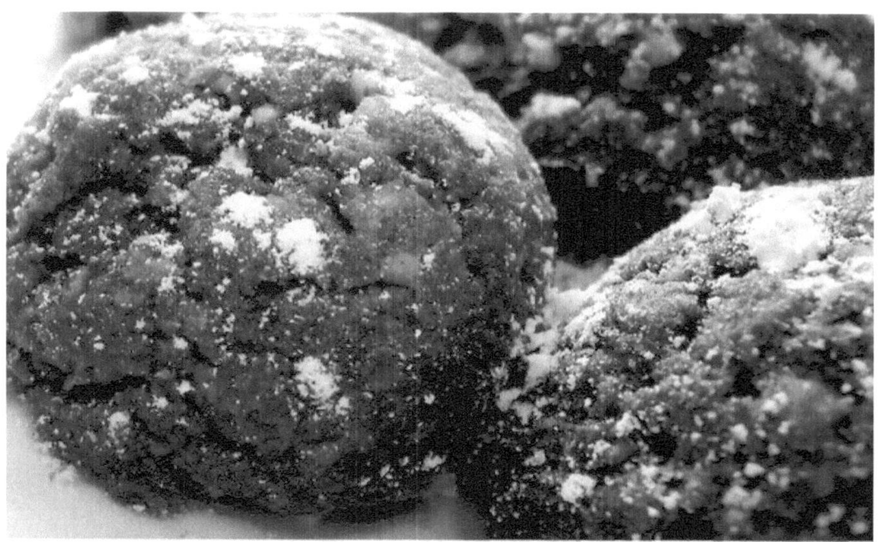

It is a quick and easy cookie recipe using pudding--pick any flavor you like!

## INGREDIENTS

- 2 tablespoons buttermilk baking mix
- 2 teaspoons vegetable oil
- 1/8 egg
- 1/8 (3.9 ounce) package instant chocolate pudding mix
- 1 tablespoon and 2-3/4 teaspoons chopped walnuts (optional)

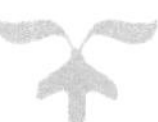

# DIRECTIONS

Servings
4

- Combine the baking mix, vegetable oil, egg and pudding mix in a bowl. Mix well. Stir in the nuts or chocolate chips (optional).
- Place teaspoonfuls on ungreased cookie sheet. Bake at 350 degrees F (175 degrees C) for 10 minutes or until toothpick comes clean.

# NUTRITION FACTS

Per Serving: 69 calories; 4.2 g total fat; 8 mg cholesterol; 140 mg sodium. 7.1 g carbohydrates; 1.1 g protein;

# CHEWY KETO CHOCOLATE COOKIES

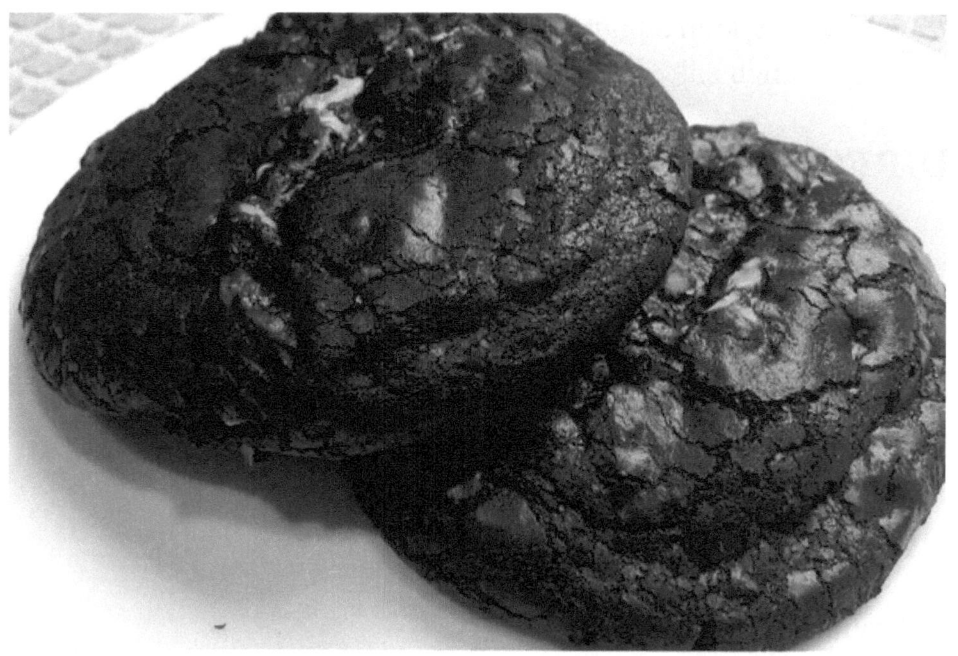

I have tried many different low-carb chocolate cookie recipes, and these are my favorite keto cookies; moist, chewy, and so decadent!

## INGREDIENTS

- 1/3 cup and 1 tablespoon almond butter
- 1/2 eggs
- 30-1/2 cups low-calorie natural sweetener (such as Swerve®)

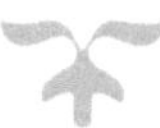

- 1 tablespoon and 1-1/4 teaspoons unsweetened cocoa powder, sifted
- 1/4 teaspoon sugar-free vanilla extract
- 1/4 pinch salt

## DIRECTIONS

Prep
10 m

Cook
12 m

Ready In
22 m

Servings
4

- Preheat oven to 350 degrees F (175 degrees C). Line a baking sheet with parchment paper.
- Combine almond butter, eggs, sweetener, cocoa powder, vanilla extract, and salt in the bowl of a food processor; pulse until a dough forms.
- Roll dough into 1-inch balls. Place on the prepared baking sheet and press down twice with a fork in a criss-cross pattern.

- Bake in the preheated oven until edges are firm, about 12 minutes. Cool on the baking sheet for 1 minute before removing to a wire rack to cool completely.

## NUTRITION FACTS

Per Serving: 173 calories; 15.7 g total fat; 25 mg cholesterol; 133 mg sodium. 12.9 g carbohydrates; 5 g protein;

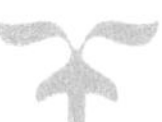

# FAUX CHOCOLATE MOUSSE

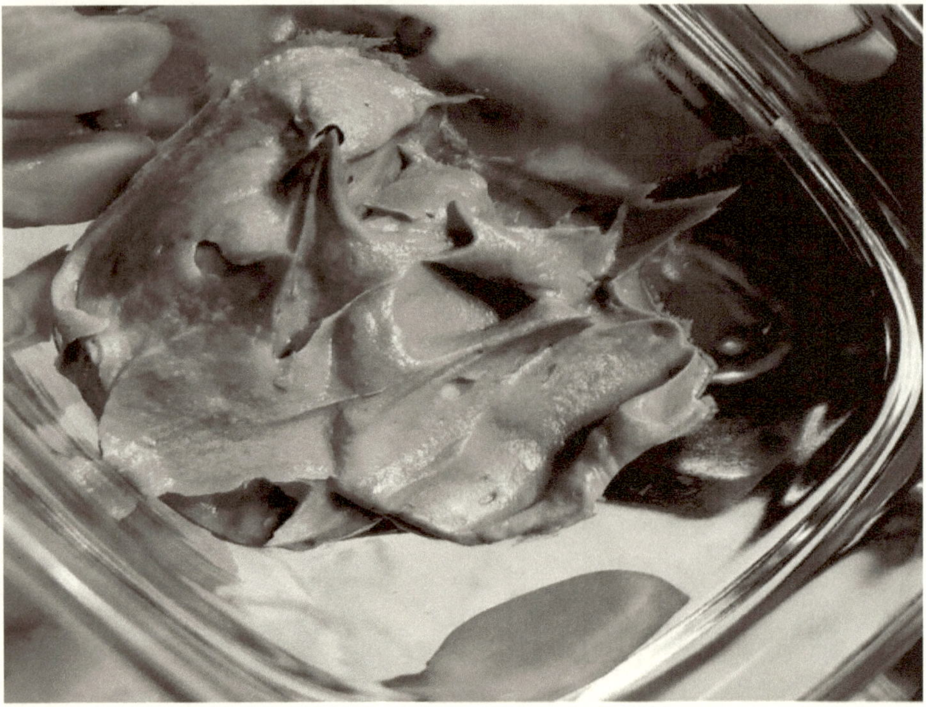

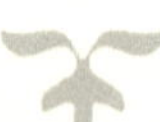

This is a quick recipe that tricks the eyes and the palate in to thinking it's authentic chocolate mousse made with cream and eggs.

## INGREDIENTS

- 1 (8 ounce) container mascarpone cheese
- 2 tablespoons heavy whipping cream

- 1 teaspoon vanilla extract
- ¼ cup chocolate chips

# DIRECTIONS

Prep
10 m

Cook
5 m

Ready In
1 hr 15 m

Servings
4

- Mix mascarpone cheese, whipping cream, and vanilla extract in a bowl.
- Melt chocolate chips in the top of a double boiler over simmering water, stirring frequently and scraping down the sides with a rubber spatula to avoid scorching.
- Fold melted chocolate into the mascarpone cheese mixture.
- Refrigerate until set, 1 to 2 hours.

# NUTRITION FACTS

Per Serving: 319 calories; 31.9 g total fat; 80 mg cholesterol; 34 mg sodium. 7 g carbohydrates; 4.6 g protein;

# PEANUT BUTTER CHOCOLATE COOKIES

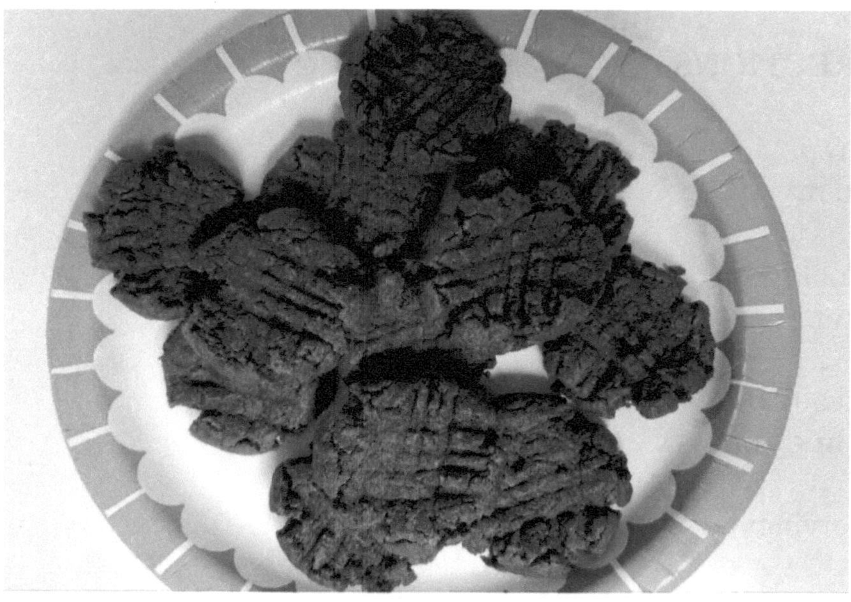

You would never guess that these tasty cookies are almost sugar free, high in protein, low carb, and gluten free. With only 5 simple ingredients you can whip these up in minutes and satisfy your peanut butter and chocolate cravings without compromising your diet! Great for low-carb, gluten-free, paleo, and keto diets!

## INGREDIENTS

- 1/4 cup creamy peanut butter
- 1/4 egg
- 9 cups stevia sweetener

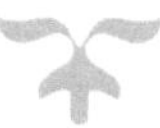

- 1-1/2 teaspoons unsweetened cocoa powder
- 3/4 teaspoon vanilla extract

## DIRECTIONS

Prep
10 m

Cook
10 m

Ready In
1 hr 55 m

Servings
4

- Preheat oven to 350 degrees F (175 degrees C).
- Combine peanut butter, egg, stevia sweetener, cocoa powder, and vanilla extract together with a mixer or food processor. Roll dough into 1-inch balls. Place 1 to 2 inches apart on an ungreased baking sheet. Flatten balls with a fork.
- Bake in the preheated oven until edges are set, about 10 minutes. Let cool on the baking sheet for 10 minutes.
- Line a tray with waxed paper. Transfer cookies to tray until cooled to room temperature, about 15 minutes, then refrigerate for 30 minutes.

# NUTRITION FACTS

Per Serving: 105 calories; 8.5 g total fat; 12 mg cholesterol; 79 mg sodium. 5.8 g carbohydrates; 4.6 g protein;

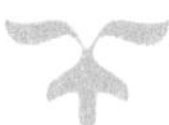

# KETO PEANUT BUTTER FUDGE FAT BOMB

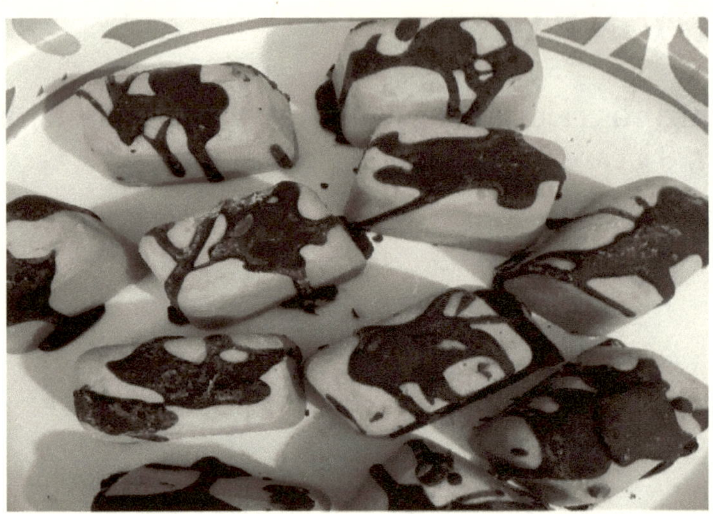

This is a great keto dessert with only 3 ingredients. If you want you can sweeten it with stevia or other sweeteners, but the peanut butter is sweet enough.

## INGREDIENTS

- 1/3 cup and 1 tablespoon unsweetened peanut butter, softened
- 1/3 cup and 1 tablespoon coconut oil
- 1 tablespoon and 1-3/4 teaspoons unsweetened vanilla-flavored almond milk
- 3-3/4 cups vanilla liquid stevia, or as needed (optional)

# DIRECTIONS

Prep
10 m

Ready In
2 hr 10 m

Servings
4

- Line a loaf pan with parchment paper.
- Combine peanut butter and coconut oil in a microwave-safe dish. Microwave 30 seconds until slightly melted. Add to blender with almond milk and stevia; blend until well combined. Pour into loaf pan and refrigerate until set, about 2 hours.

# NUTRITION FACTS

Per Serving: 341 calories; 34.9 g total fat; 0 mg cholesterol; 122 mg sodium. 5.3 g carbohydrates; 6.5 g protein;

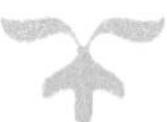

# DRINKS

## GREEN LEMONADE

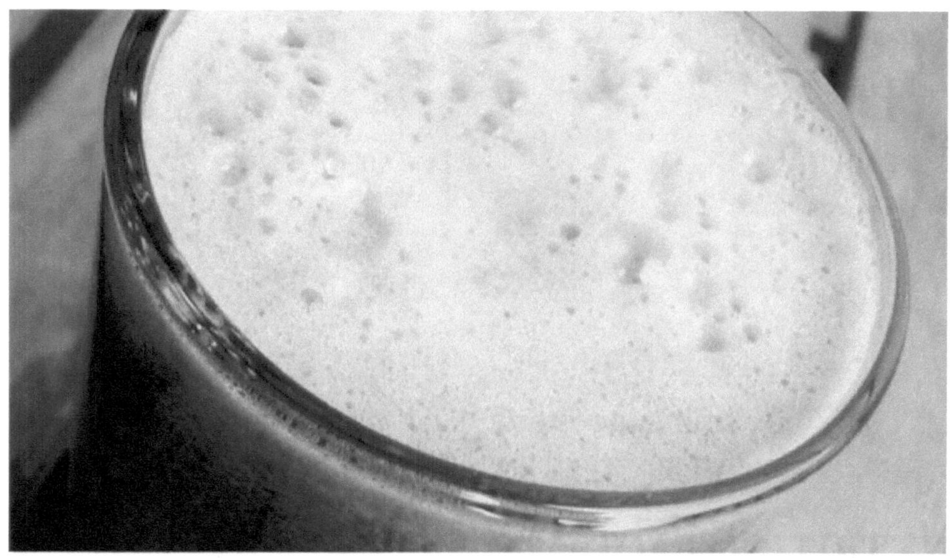

"This drink requires a juicer to make. It is super healthy and loaded with powerful nutrition."

## INGREDIENTS

- 1 head romaine lettuce
- 4 leaves kale
- 1 (1/2 inch) piece ginger
- 2 apples, quartered
- 1 lemon

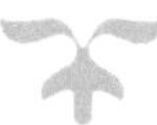

# DIRECTIONS

Prep
10 m

Ready In
10 m

Servings
1

- Process romaine lettuce, kale, ginger, apples, and lemon through a juicer. Stir before drinking.

## NUTRITION FACTS

Per Serving: 265 calories; 2.4 g fat; 69.7 g carbohydrates; 8.9 g protein; 0 mg cholesterol; 68 mg sodium.

# HONEY LEMON TEA

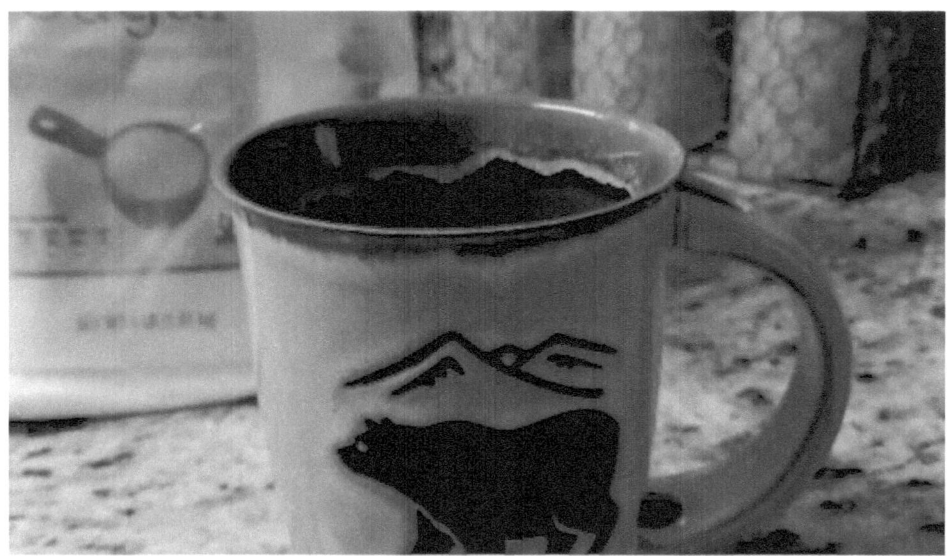

Suffering from a cold? Warm your body and soothe your throat with a hot cup of Honey and Lemon Tea! It's the perfect cold remedy.

## INGREDIENTS

- 1 cup water
- 2 teaspoons honey
- 1 teaspoon fresh lemon juice
- 1 teaspoon white sugar, or to taste

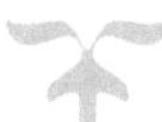

# DIRECTIONS

Prep
1 m

Cook
2 m

Ready In
3 m

Servings
1

- Pour water into a mug. Add honey and heat in the microwave for 1 minute and 30 seconds. Stir in lemon juice, mixing until honey is dissolved, then stir in the sugar.

# NUTRITION FACTS

Per Serving: 63 calories; 0 g fat; 16.9 g carbohydrates; 0.1 g protein; 0 mg cholesterol; < 1 mg sodium.

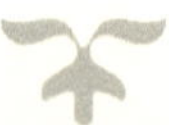

# FRIENDSHIP TEA

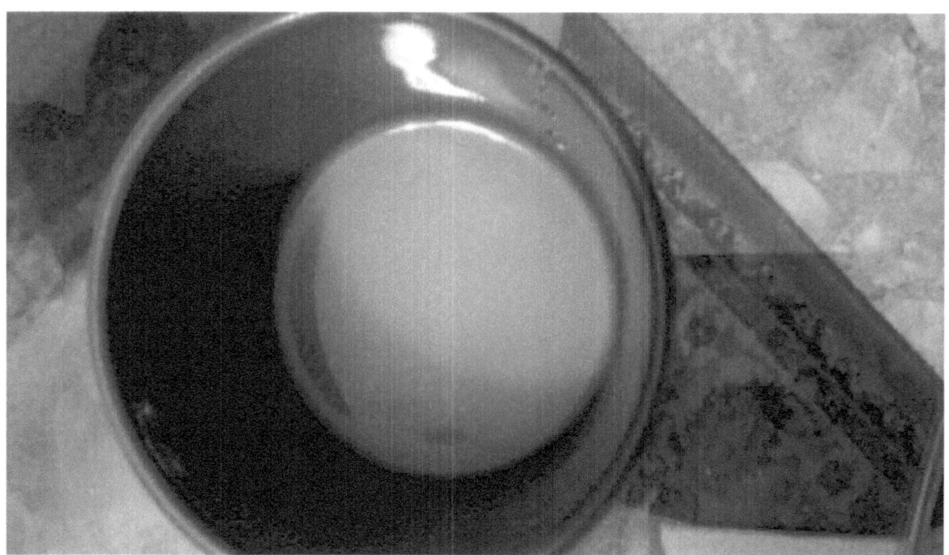

"This is a lemony spiced tea mix with cinnamon and clove that makes great gifts during the holidays, or any time!"

## INGREDIENTS

- 1/2 cup instant tea powder
- 1 cup sweetened lemonade powder
- 1 cup orange-flavored drink mix (e.g. Tang)
- 1 teaspoon ground cinnamon
- 1/2 teaspoon ground cloves

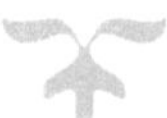

# DIRECTIONS

Prep
10 m

Ready In
10 m

Servings
1

- In a large bowl, combine instant tea, lemonade powder, orange drink mix, cinnamon and clove. Mix well and store in an airtight container.
- To serve, Put 2 to 3 teaspoons of mix in a mug. Stir in 1 cup of boiling water. Adjust to taste.

# NUTRITION FACTS

Per Serving: 39 calories; 0 g fat; 9.9 g carbohydrates; 0.1 g protein; 0 mg cholesterol; 2 mg sodium.

# SMOOTH SWEET TEA

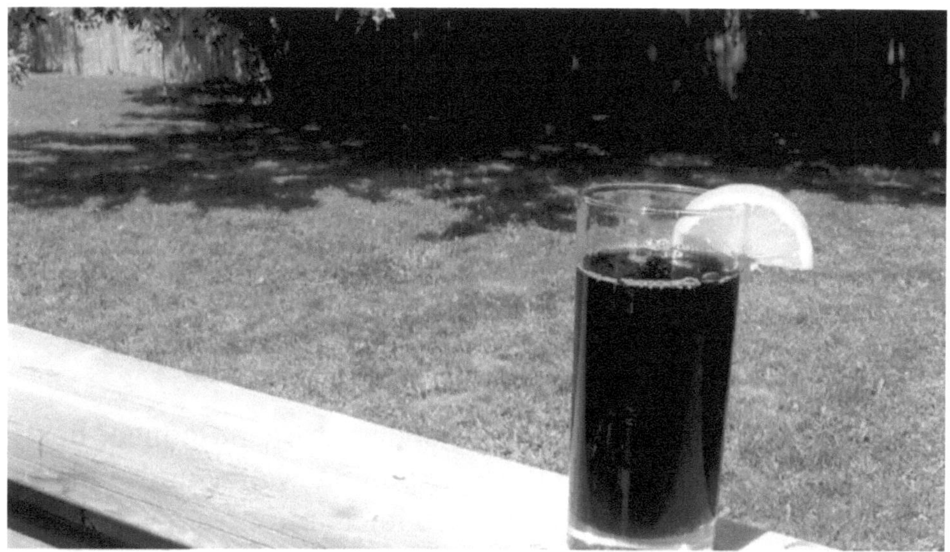

"Southern sweet tea, perfect for hot summer days!"

## INGREDIENTS

- 1 pinch baking soda
- 2 cups boiling water
- 6 tea bags
- 3/4 cup white sugar
- 6 cups cool water

## DIRECTIONS

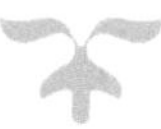

Prep
5 m

Cook
15 m

Ready In
3 h 20 m

Servings
8

- Sprinkle a pinch of baking soda into a 64-ounce, heat-proof, glass pitcher. Pour in boiling water, and add tea bags. Cover, and allow to steep for 15 minutes.
- Remove tea bags, and discard; stir in sugar until dissolved. Pour in cool water, then refrigerate until cold.

## NUTRITION FACTS

Per Serving: 73 calories; 0 g fat; 18.7 g carbohydrates; 0 g protein; 0 mg cholesterol; 41 mg sodium.

## ICED LEMON COFFEE

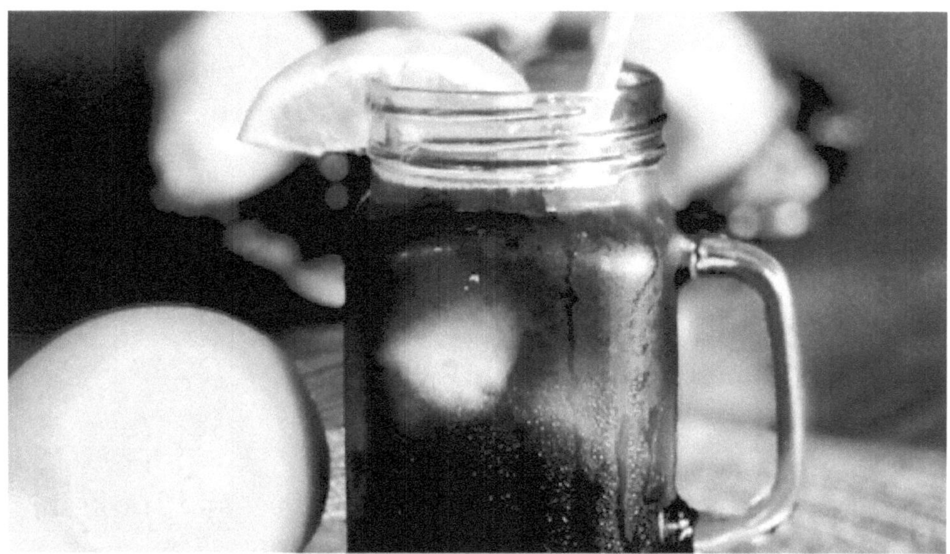

Brighten your brew with lemonade and a splash of sparkling water, It may seem an unlikely combination, but adding lemonade to your iced coffee creates a bold, tangy and delicious drink. Think of it as an Arnold Palmer, with strong coffee instead of black tea.

## INGREDIENTS

- 1 cup cold-brewed coffee
- 1/4 cup ice cubes
- 1/4 cup freshly squeezed lemon juice
- 1 teaspoon stevia powder, or to taste

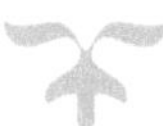

- 1 slice lemon, for garnish

# DIRECTIONS

Prep
5 m

Ready In
5 m

Servings
1

- Combine coffee, ice cubes, lemon juice, and stevia in a glass. Stir. Garnish with a slice of lemon.

# NUTRITION FACTS

Per Serving: 23 calories; 0.1 g fat; 9.6 g carbohydrates; 0.7 g protein; 0 mg cholesterol; 6 mg sodium.

# PALEO AND KETO ALMOND BUTTER MOCHA FOR TWO

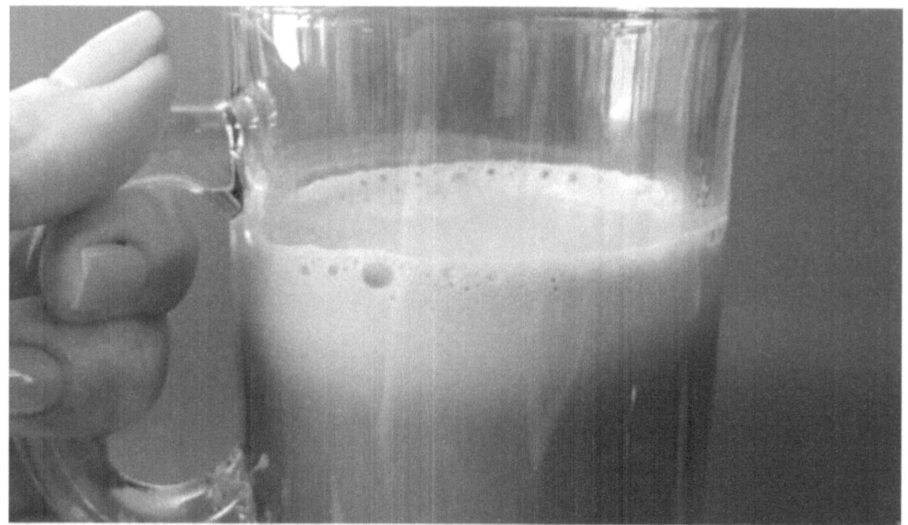

"This low-carb rich and decadent almond butter mocha will keep you fueled all day! It is ideal for keto and Paleo diets."

## INGREDIENTS

- 1 1/2 cups warm almond milk
- 1 tablespoon almond butter
- 2 tablespoons instant espresso powder
- 1 tablespoon unsweetened cocoa powder
- 1/2 teaspoon vanilla extract
- 1/2 teaspoon stevia powder

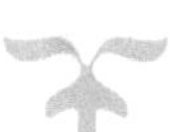

# DIRECTIONS

Prep
10 m

Ready In
10 m

Servings
1

- Combine almond milk, almond butter, espresso powder, cocoa powder, vanilla extract, and stevia powder in a blender; mix until well combined and slightly thickened, about 2 minutes. Serve in 2 mugs; dust with cocoa powder.

# NUTRITION FACTS

Per Serving: 115 calories; 7.1 g fat; 11.5 g carbohydrates; 2.8 g protein; 0 mg cholesterol; 157 mg sodium.

# BREAKFAST ZINGER JUICE

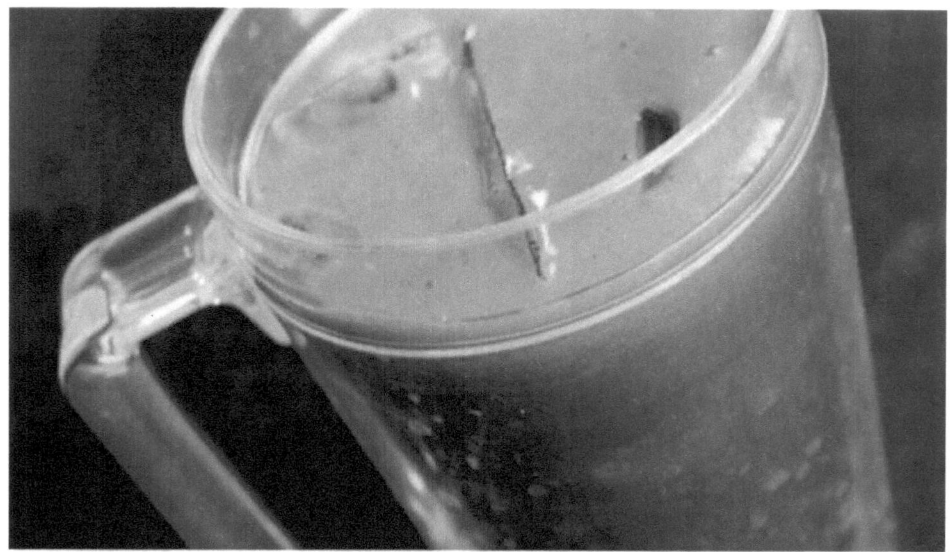

"This is a delicious, cleansing juice that's great in the morning. Great way to kick start your day, while getting necessary vitamins."

## INGREDIENTS

- 2 lemons - peeled, seeded, and quartered
- 2 carrots, chopped
- 2 apples, quartered
- 2 beets, trimmed and chopped

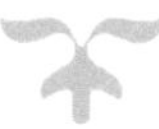

# DIRECTIONS

Prep
5 m

Ready In
5 m

Servings
1

- Press lemons, carrots, apples, and beets through a juicer and into a large glass.

# NUTRITION FACTS

Per Serving: 158 calories; 0.9 g fat; 45.4 g carbohydrates; 3.6 g protein; 0 mg cholesterol; 118 mg sodium.

# CARROT AND ORANGE JUICE

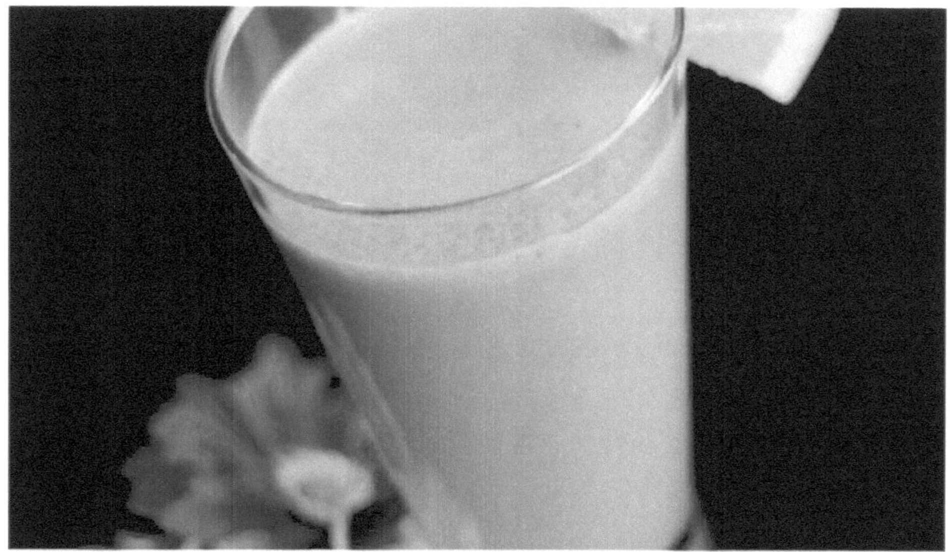

"This quick, fresh, and delicious juice is one of my favorite morning drinks!"

## INGREDIENTS

- 2 pounds organic carrots, trimmed and scrubbed
- 8 organic oranges, peeled

## DIRECTIONS

Prep
10 m

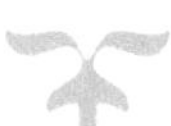

Ready In
10 m

Servings
1

- Press carrots and oranges through a juicer and into a large glass.

## NUTRITION FACTS

Per Serving: 183 calories; 0.8 g fat; 44.3 g carbohydrates; 3.9 g protein; 0 mg cholesterol; 157 mg sodium.

# BREAKFAST IN BANGKOK

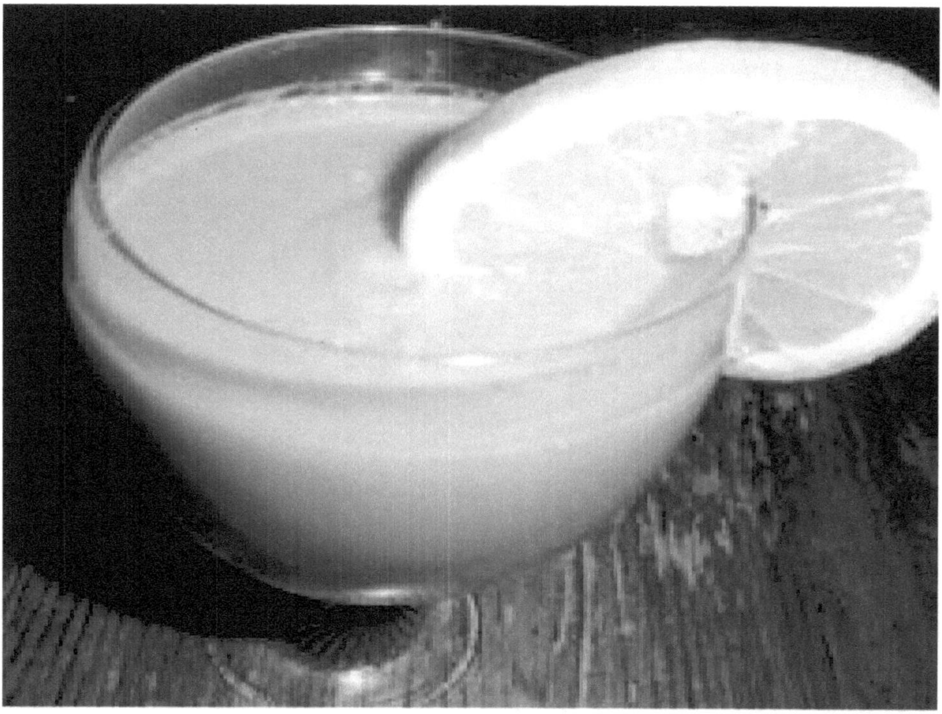

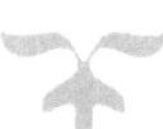

"Deliriously delicious juice to start your day! The result will be a lovely, creamy, silky smooth beverage - and with a lovely orange glow, it's a real eye catcher, too!"

## INGREDIENTS

- 2 carrots
- 1 Gala apple, peeled and quartered

- 1/4 cup coconut milk
- 1/4 teaspoon grated fresh ginger root

## DIRECTIONS

Prep
5 m

Ready In
5 m

Servings
1

- Run the carrots and apple through a juice extractor and pour the resulting juice into a glass. Stir in the coconut milk and garnish with freshly grated ginger root.

## NUTRITION FACTS

Per Serving: 242 calories; 12.6 g fat; 34.5 g carbohydrates; 2.8 g protein; 0 mg cholesterol; 108 mg sodium.

## BEER MARGARITAS

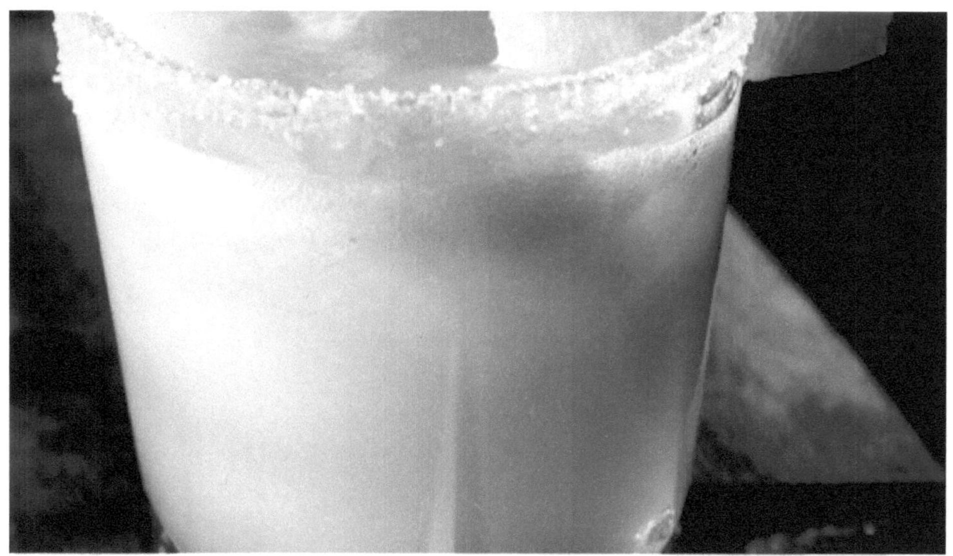

"Who would believe that beer would be the perfect solution to eradicating fluorescent green margaritas? Well, it is! Best to use not-so-micro brews to avoid an overpowering beer flavor. Use the limeade can to measure the ingredients, and adjust with extra water if the mixture seems too sweet. Straining the pulp is always a good idea, unless, of course, you like pulp!"

# INGREDIENTS

- 1 (12 fluid ounce) can frozen limeade concentrate
- 12 fluid ounces tequila
- 12 fluid ounces water

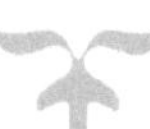

- 12 fluid ounces beer
- ice
- 1 lime, cut into wedges

# DIRECTIONS

Prep
5 m

Ready In
5 m

Servings
1

- Pour limeade, tequila, water, and beer into a large pitcher. Stir until well-blended, and limeade has melted. Add plenty of ice, and garnish with lime wedges. Adjust with additional water, if needed.

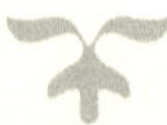

# FUSS FREE HOT CRANBERRY TEA

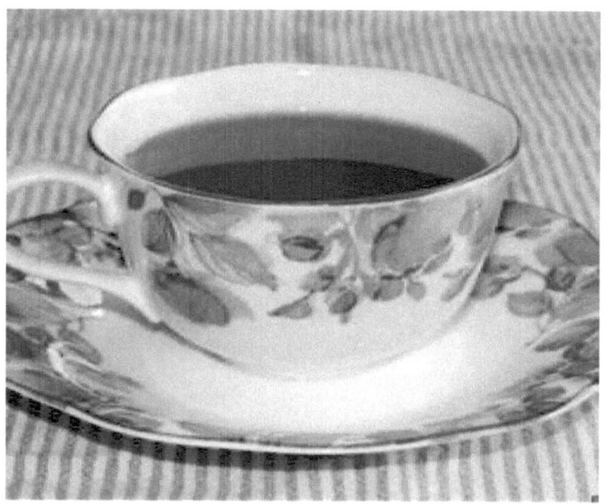

I have looked for recipes for hot cranberry tea that are simple and don't involve a lot of time.

## INGREDIENTS

- 1/2 gallon orange juice
- 1 (64 fluid ounce) bottle cranberry-raspberry juice
- 1 (16 ounce) can pineapple juice
- 2 (2.25 ounce) packages small red cinnamon candies
- 1/2 gallon water
- 8 tea bags

# DIRECTIONS

Prep
5 m

Cook
10 m

Ready In
15 m

Servings
26

- Combine the orange juice, cranberry-raspberry juice, pineapple juice, and cinnamon candies in a large stockpot; cook over high heat until the candies dissolve.
- Combine the water and tea bags in a separate pot and bring to a boil; reduce heat and simmer 5 to 10 minutes; pour into juice mixture. Serve hot.

# NUTRITION FACTS

Per Serving: 100 calories; 0.2 g fat; 24.3 g carbohydrates; 0.6 g protein; 0 mg cholesterol; 7 mg sodium.

# WATERMELON AGUA FRESCA

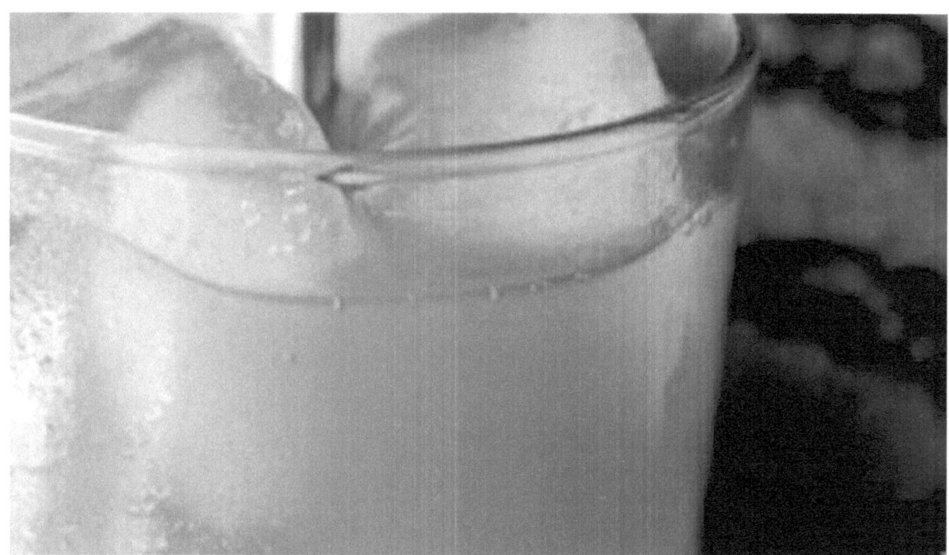

"This is my all-time favorite summertime drink. When it's hot and humid and you're totally parched, there's nothing as refreshing, as revitalizing, and as restorative as ice-cold watermelon agua fresca. It's one of life's great drinkable pleasures."

## INGREDIENTS

- 1/2 seedless watermelon
- 2 cups cold water
- 1/2 cup white sugar, or to taste
- 1/2 cup water

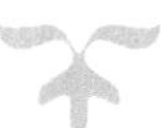

# DIRECTIONS

Prep
10 m

Ready In
50 m

Servings
6

- Scoop flesh from watermelon half and transfer watermelon to a blender. Add 2 cups cold water. Place a folded towel on blender lid and blend until liquefied, about 1 minute. Strain through a fine mesh strainer into a large bowl to remove fibers. Discard fibers left in strainer. Skim and discard excess foam from juice if desired.
- Place sugar and 1/2 cup water into a saucepan over medium heat and stir until water is hot and sugar has dissolved. Turn off heat and let simple syrup cool to room temperature. Stir simple syrup into watermelon juice to taste.
- Pour drink into a 2-quart pitcher and refrigerate until cold, at least 30 minutes. To serve, fill tall glasses with ice cubes and pour agua fresca drink over ice. Serve with straws.

# NUTRITION FACTS

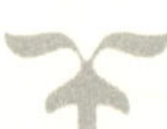

Per Serving: 177 calories; 0.6 g fat; 45 g carbohydrates; 2.3 g protein; 0 mg cholesterol; 7 mg sodium.

# CELYNE'S GREEN JUICE

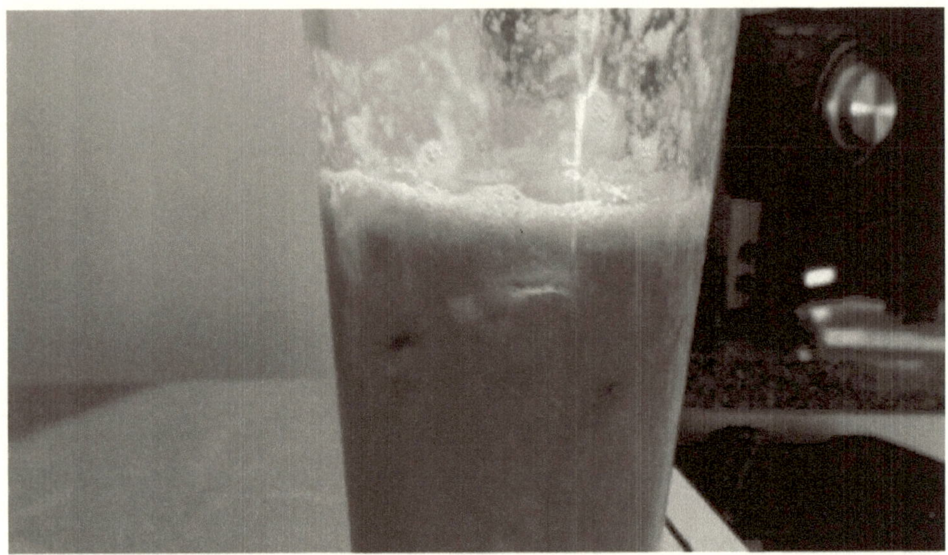

Great juicer recipe with veggies you won't taste. Great for kids as they don't taste the veggies

## INGREDIENTS

- 2 oranges, peeled
- 1 lemon, peeled
- 1 green apple, quartered
- 1 cup fresh spinach
- 1 leaf kale

# DIRECTIONS

Prep
10 m

Ready In
10 m

Servings
1

- Process oranges, lemon, green apple, spinach, and kale through a juicer according to manufacturer's recommendations.

# NUTRITION FACTS

Per Serving: 44 calories; 0.2 g fat; 11.1 g carbohydrates; 0.9 g protein; 0 mg cholesterol; 17 mg sodium.

# SIMPLE SYRUP

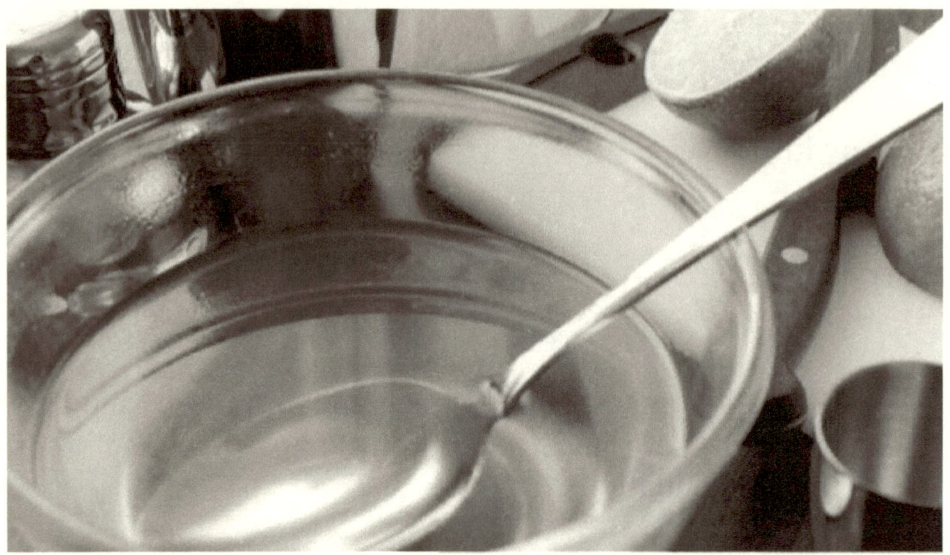

"Simple syrup is a commonly used ingredient in many cocktails and other drink recipes. It's also easy to make!"

## INGREDIENTS

- 1 cup white sugar
- 1 cup water

## DIRECTIONS

Prep
1 m

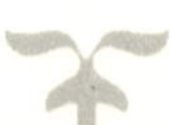

Cook
10 m

Ready In
30 m

Servings
1

- In a medium saucepan combine sugar and water. Bring to a boil, stirring, until sugar has dissolved. Allow to cool.

## NUTRITION FACTS

Per Serving: 48 calories; 0 g fat; 12.5 g carbohydrates; 0 g protein; 0 mg cholesterol; < 1 mg sodium.

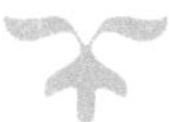

## BEVERAGE CUBES

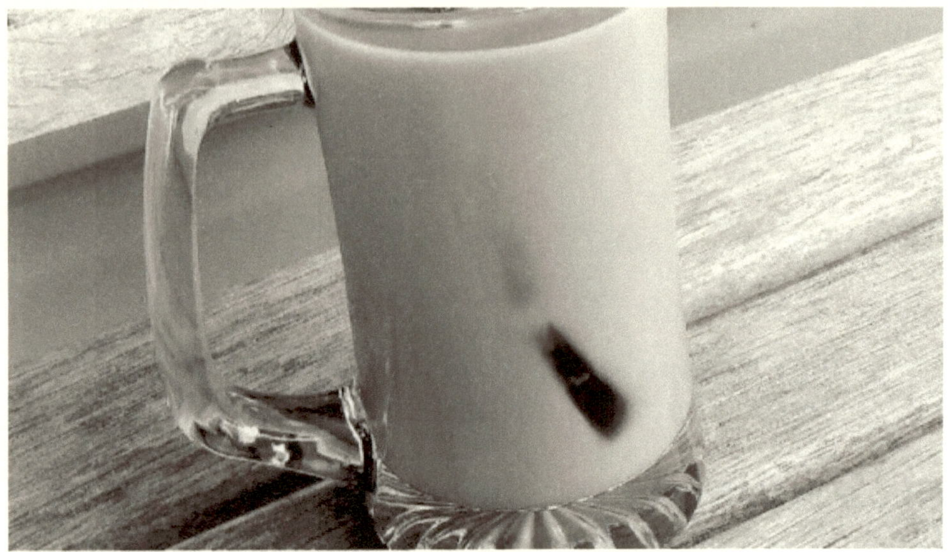

"Everyone has a favorite drink that is always in the fridge...but don't you hate it when your ice cubes melt and make your drink watery? Here's a simple solution! Use your favorite non-carbonated beverage; fruit juice, coffee and prepared drink mix all work great."

## INGREDIENTS

- 2 cups brewed black tea, cold

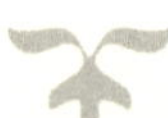

# DIRECTIONS

Prep
1 m

Ready In
1 m

Servings
12

- Pour the cold tea into an ice cube tray and freeze. Pop out a few whenever you're ready for a tall cool drink.

# NUTRITION FACTS

Per Serving: < 1 calories; 0 g fat; 0.1 g carbohydrates; 0 g protein; 0 mg cholesterol; 1 mg sodium.

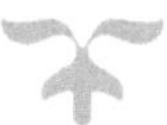

# BOSTON ICED TEA

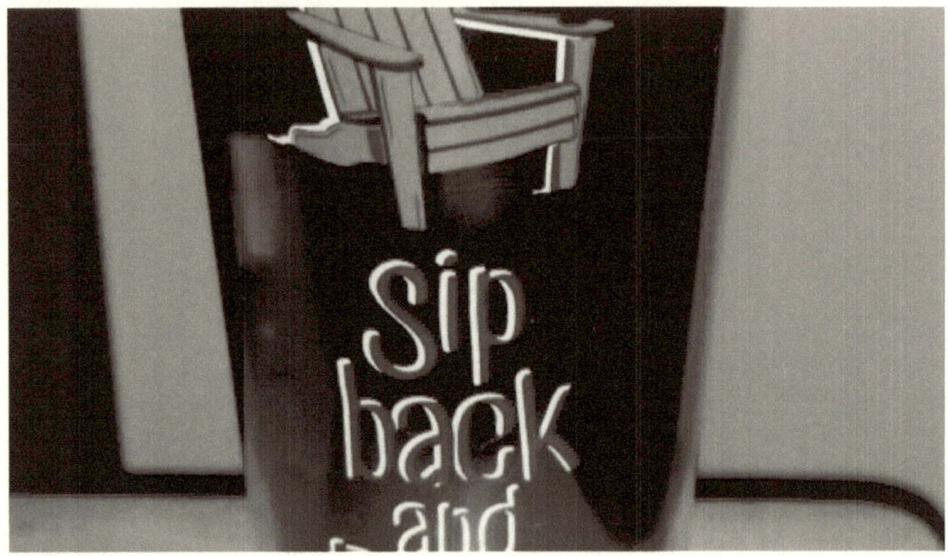


When you think of Boston and tea, you probably think of the Boston Tea Party. But the city links to tea in another way – Boston Iced Tea, which combines tea with cranberry juice.

## INGREDIENTS

- 1 gallon water
- 1 cup white sugar
- 15 tea bags
- 1 (12 fluid ounce) can frozen cranberry juice concentrate

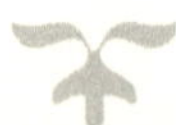

# DIRECTIONS

Prep
20 m

Cook
15 m

Ready In
35 m

Servings
14

- Put water in large pot, and heat on high until boiling. Add sugar and stir until dissolved. Add teabags and let steep until desired strength is acquired. Stir in cranberry juice concentrate, and allow to cool.

## NUTRITION FACTS

Per Serving: 118 calories; 0 g fat; 30.3 g carbohydrates; 0 g protein; 0 mg cholesterol; 9 mg sodium.

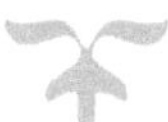

# ORANGE SPICE TEA MIX

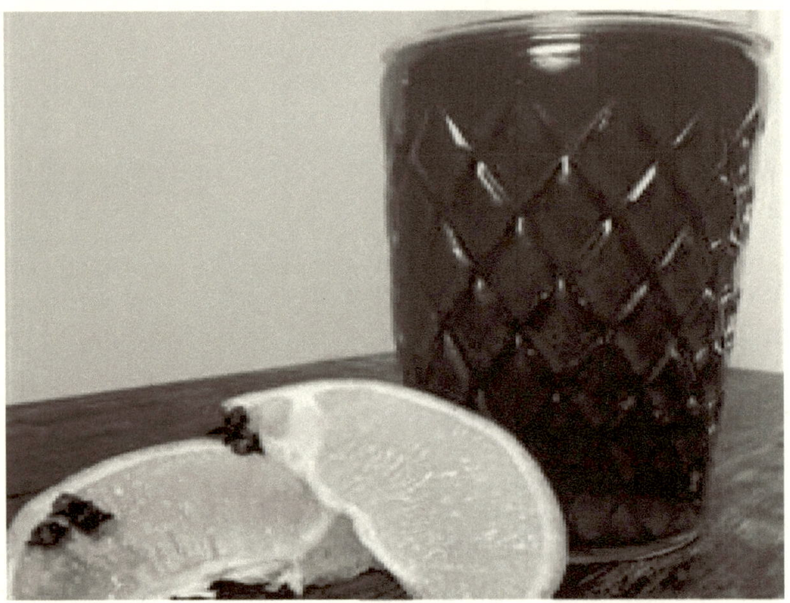

"A nice spicy tea mixture that can be given as a gift."

## INGREDIENTS

- 1 cinnamon stick, broken into pieces
- 5 whole cloves
- 2 tablespoons dried orange peel
- 2 whole black peppercorns
- 6 black tea bags, strings removed

# DIRECTIONS

Prep
10 m

Ready In
10 m

Servings
8

- In a small bowl, combine cinnamon stick, cloves, orange peel and peppercorns. Place spice mixture and the tea bags in a cheesecloth bag, and tie with kitchen string.
- To prepare tea: Bring 8 cups water to boil. Add cheesecloth bag and steep for 5 minutes.

# NUTRITION FACTS

Per Serving: 9 calories; 0.1 g fat; 2.1 g carbohydrates; 0.2 g protein; 0 mg cholesterol; 2 mg sodium.

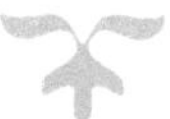

# WATERMELON AND BELL PEPPER SLUSH

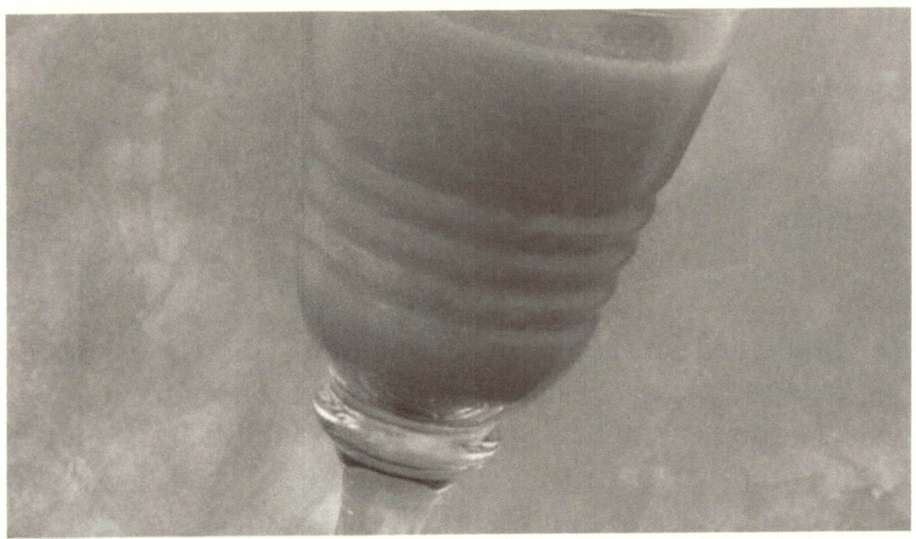

"Light, refreshing, and super simple. It's naturally sweet and a perfect treat for a summer day. Actually, they sell the same exact thing in a tourist town in Florida for $5 a glass! Use sweet red, orange, or yellow bell peppers."

## INGREDIENTS

- 3 cups cubed seeded watermelon
- 1/2 red bell pepper, seeded and coarsely chopped
- 3 cups ice
- 1 sprig fresh mint

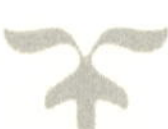

# DIRECTIONS

Prep
10 m

Ready In
10 m

Servings
4

- Place the watermelon, red bell pepper, and ice in a blender, and blend until the ice is crushed and the drink is slushy. Pour into glasses, and garnish with fresh mint leaves. Can be stored in refrigerator up to 2 days.

# NUTRITION FACTS

Per Serving: 40 calories; 0.2 g fat; 9.7 g carbohydrates; 0.9 g protein; 0 mg cholesterol; 7 mg sodium.

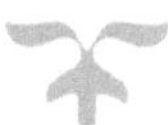

# INSTANT RUSSIAN TEA

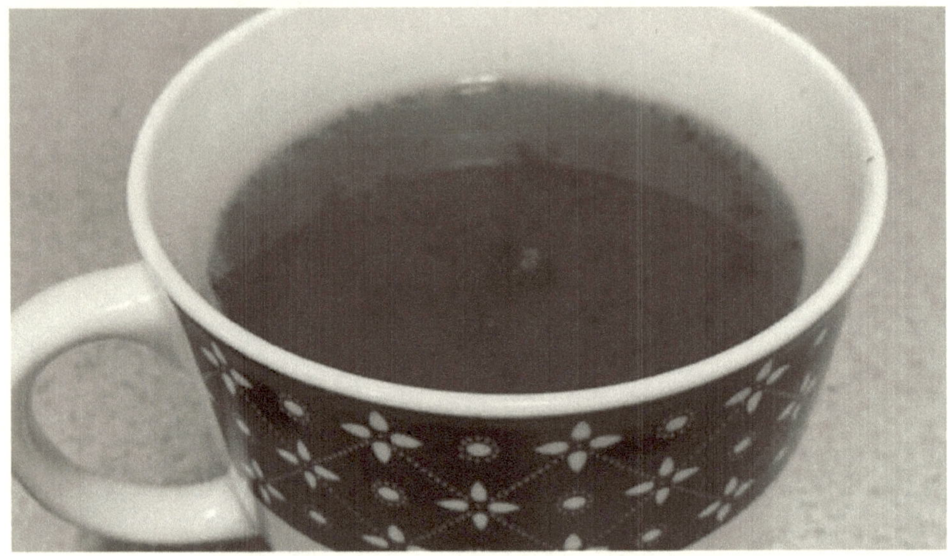

Instant Russian Tea recipe with Tang is an old holiday favorite that's the perfect inexpensive hot drink for the holidays!

## INGREDIENTS

- 2 cups orange-flavored drink mix (e.g. Tang)
- 2 cups white sugar
- 1/4 cup instant tea powder
- 3/4 cup lemon-flavored instant tea powder
- 1 teaspoon ground cinnamon
- 1 teaspoon ground cloves

# DIRECTIONS

Prep
10 m

Ready In
10 m

Servings
100

In a large bowl, combine orange drink mix, sugar, tea powder, cinnamon and cloves. Mix well and store in an airtight container.
To serve, put 3 teaspoons of mix in a mug. Stir in 1 cup boiling water. Adjust to taste.

# NUTRITION FACTS

Per Serving: 32 calories; 0 g fat; 8.4 g carbohydrates; 0.1 g protein; 0 mg cholesterol; < 1 mg sodium.

# CUCUMBER COOLER

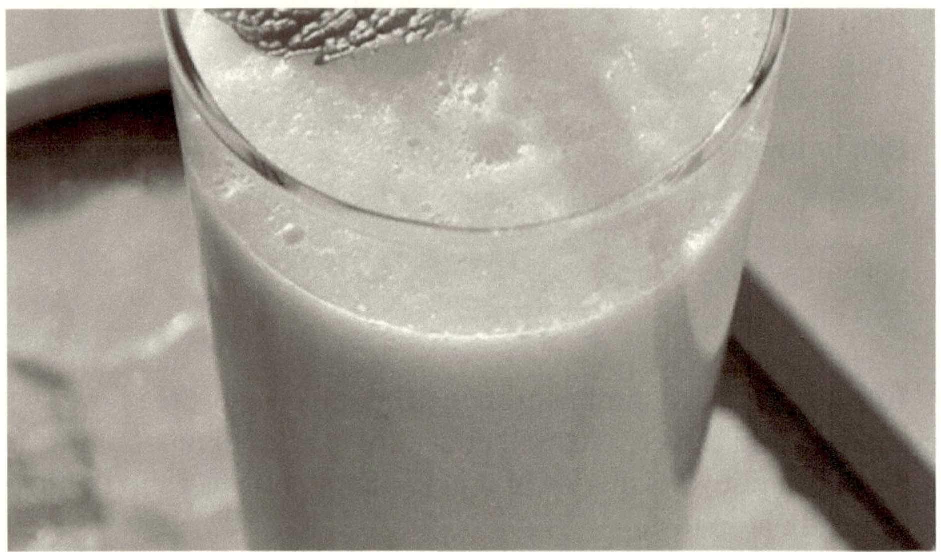

There's no alcohol in our recipe for a cucumber drink flavored with mashed mint leaves and lime, but this lightly sweet beverage is more refreshing than any cocktail.

## INGREDIENTS

- 2 cucumbers - peeled, seeded, and chopped
- 3/8 cup fresh lime juice
- 1/3 cup white sugar
- 2/3 cup water

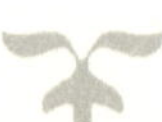

# DIRECTIONS

Prep
10 m

Ready In
10 m

Servings
4

- Combine the cucumber, lime juice, sugar, and water in a food processor; puree.

# NUTRITION FACTS

Per Serving: 365 calories; 0.7 g fat; 94.8 g carbohydrates; 4 g protein; 0 mg cholesterol; 18 mg sodium.

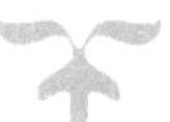

## SPICED TEA MIX

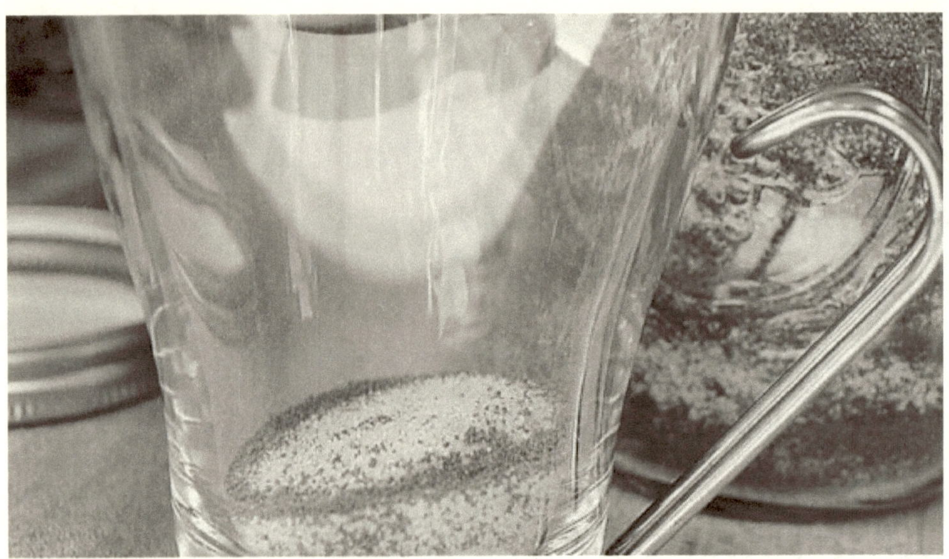

"This is a delicious dry spiced tea mix which can be packed in jars and given as gifts. It can also be prepared sugar free by using sugar free orange flavored drink mix and sugar free iced tea mix."

## INGREDIENTS

- 1 (3 ounce) package lemon-flavored ice tea mix
- 2 (1.8 ounce) packages orange-flavored drink mix
- 1 1/3 tablespoons ground cinnamon
- 2 teaspoons ground cloves

# DIRECTIONS

Servings
6

- Combine iced tea mix, orange flavored drink mix, ground cinnamon, and ground cloves. Store in an airtight container.
- To serve, stir 1 1/2 teaspoon mix into 1 cup hot water.

## NUTRITION FACTS

Per Serving: 116 calories; 0.2 g fat; 29.2 g carbohydrates; 1.1 g protein; 0 mg cholesterol; 11 mg sodium.

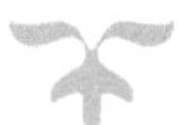

# CUCUMBER TEA SPRITZER

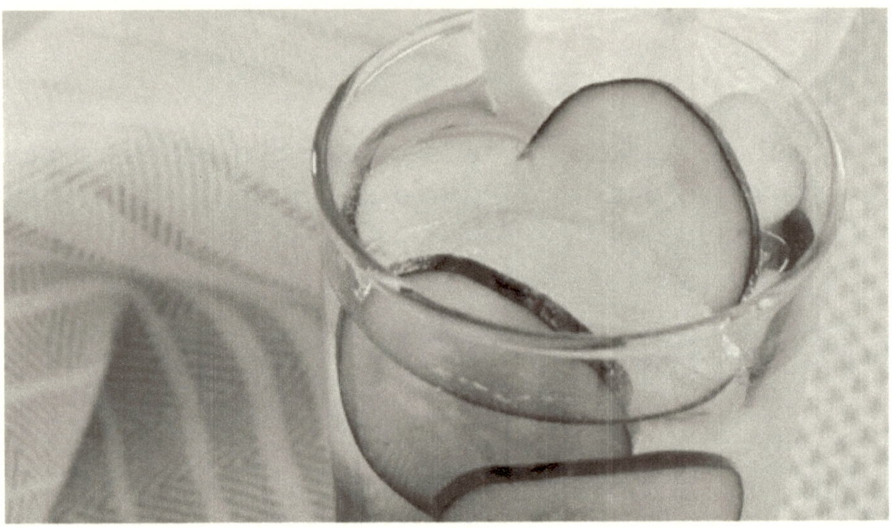

"A great summer drink or just a nice refreshing mocktail - cucumber water is healthy too!"

## INGREDIENTS

- 2 cups water
- 1/2 cup white sugar
- 2 black tea bags, or more to taste
- ice
- 1 cucumber, cut into 1/4-inch slices
- 5 cups sparkling water, or as needed
- 1 lemon

# DIRECTIONS

Prep
10 m

Cook
5 m

Ready In
20 m

Servings
5

- Bring water to a boil in a kettle. Pour into a pitcher. Stir in sugar until it dissolves into a syrup. Add tea bags; let steep, about 5 minutes.
- Fill 5 glasses with ice cubes. Add some cucumber slices. Fill glasses 3/4 full of sparking water. Divide sweet tea evenly among glasses. Squeeze some lemon juice into each drink; stir.

## NUTRITION FACTS

Per Serving: 83 calories; 0 g fat; 21.4 g carbohydrates; 0.3 g protein; 0 mg cholesterol; 23 mg sodium.

# THAI ICED TEA (CHA YEN)

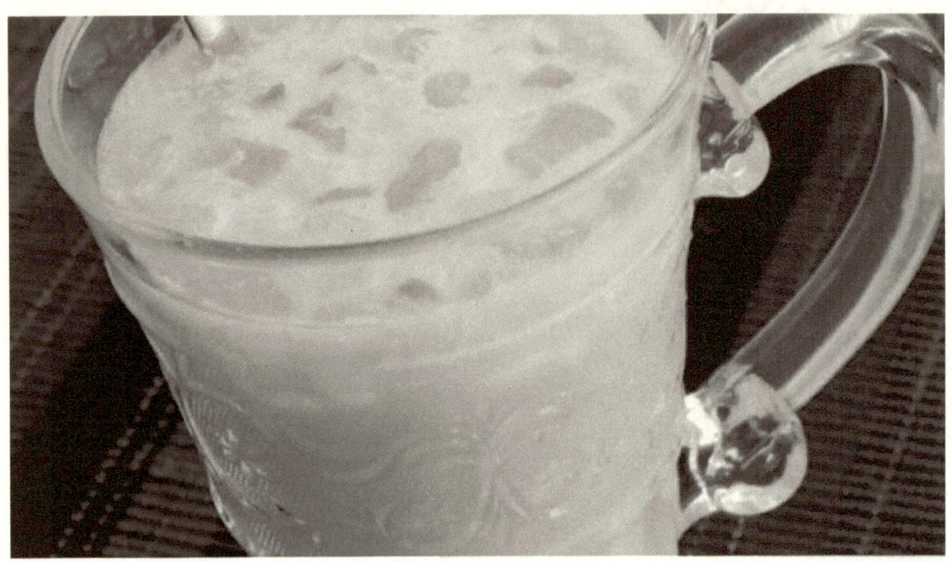

"A drink that is starting to gain popularity. Almost like a latte but made with tea. My husband loves this."

## INGREDIENTS

- 1 cup water
- 2 1/2 tablespoons black tea leaves
- 4 1/2 tablespoons white sugar
- 1/4 cup evaporated milk
- crushed ice
- 1 tablespoon milk, divided (optional)

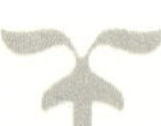

# DIRECTIONS

Prep
5 m

Cook
15 m

Ready In
20 m

Servings
2

- Bring water to a boil in a small saucepan. Remove from heat and add black tea; let steep about 10 minutes or to desired strength.
- Strain tea into a container and discard leaves. Add sugar and evaporated milk; stir until sugar is dissolved.
- Fill 2 glasses with ice. Pour tea over ice. Top each glass with 1 1/2 teaspoon milk.

## NUTRITION FACTS

Per Serving: 159 calories; 2.6 g fat; 31.8 g carbohydrates; 3.1 g protein; 10 mg cholesterol; 42 mg sodium.

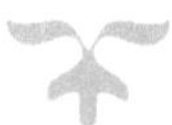

# COCOA TEA MIX RECIPE

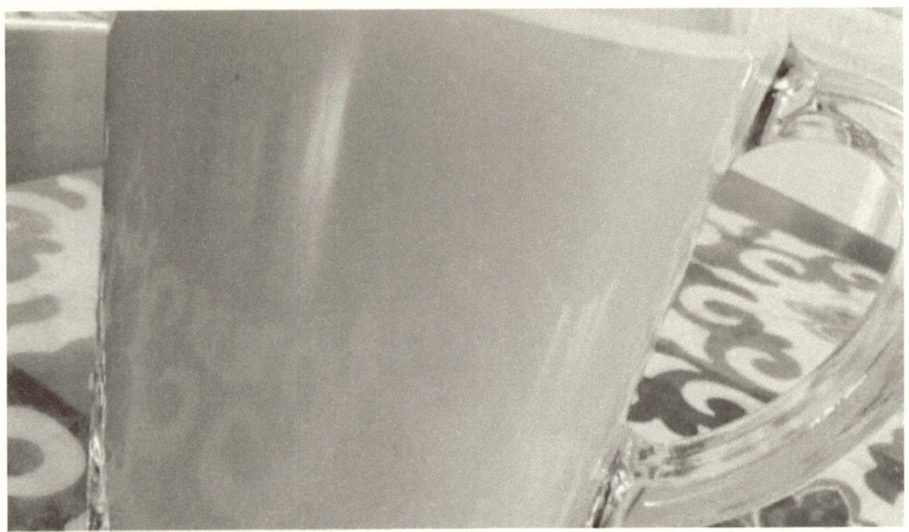

"Not everyone will be a fan of this earthy, sweet drink. Depends what tea you use really."

## INGREDIENTS

- 1 1/2 cups boiling water
- 1 Earl Grey tea bag
- 3 tablespoons milk
- 1 1/2 tablespoons hot cocoa mix
- 2 teaspoons white sugar

# DIRECTIONS

Prep
10 m

Ready In
10 m

Servings
1

- Pour boiling water into a mug and steep tea bag, about 2 minutes. Remove tea bag; add milk, hot cocoa mix, and sugar. Stir until well-blended, about 20 seconds.

# NUTRITION FACTS

Per Serving: 103 calories; 1.4 g fat; 20.5 g carbohydrates; 2.3 g protein; 4 mg cholesterol; 90 mg sodium.

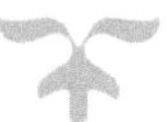

# WATERMELON SUMMERTIME SLUSH

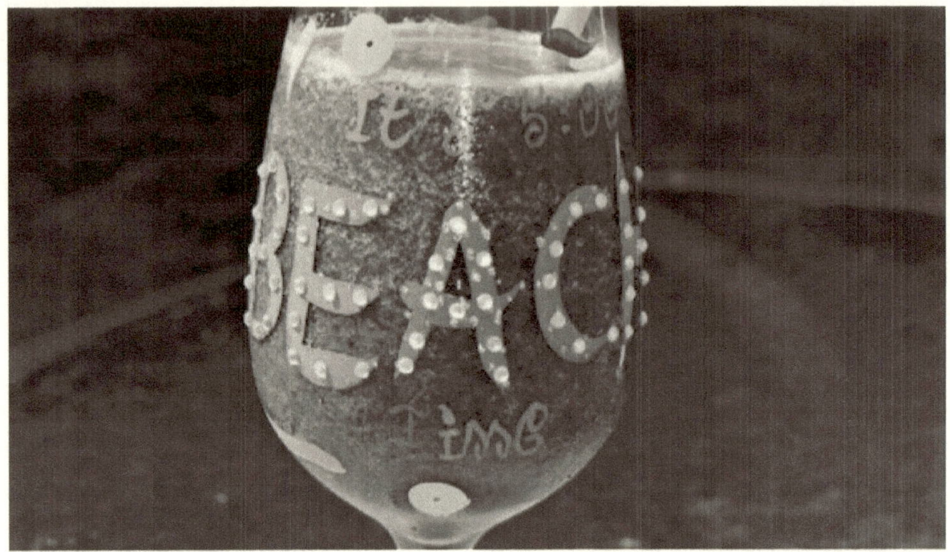

"A crisp and refreshing summertime treat! This drink is a great afternoon pick-me-up."

## INGREDIENTS

- 1 cup ice cubes
- 1/2 cup coconut water (liquid from inside coconut)
- 1/4 cup cherries, pitted
- 1 cup cubed, seeded watermelon
- 1 teaspoon granular sucralose sweetener (optional)

# DIRECTIONS

Prep
10 m

Ready In
10 m

Servings
2

- Place ice in a blender and pour in coconut water; add cherries, watermelon cubes, and sweetener. Cover and blend until slushy, about 1 minute. Pour into 2 glasses to serve.

## NUTRITION FACTS

Per Serving: 48 calories; 0.4 g fat; 11 g carbohydrates; 1.1 g protein; 0 mg cholesterol; 67 mg sodium.

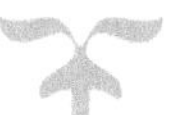

# CHOCOLATE-Y ICED MOCHA

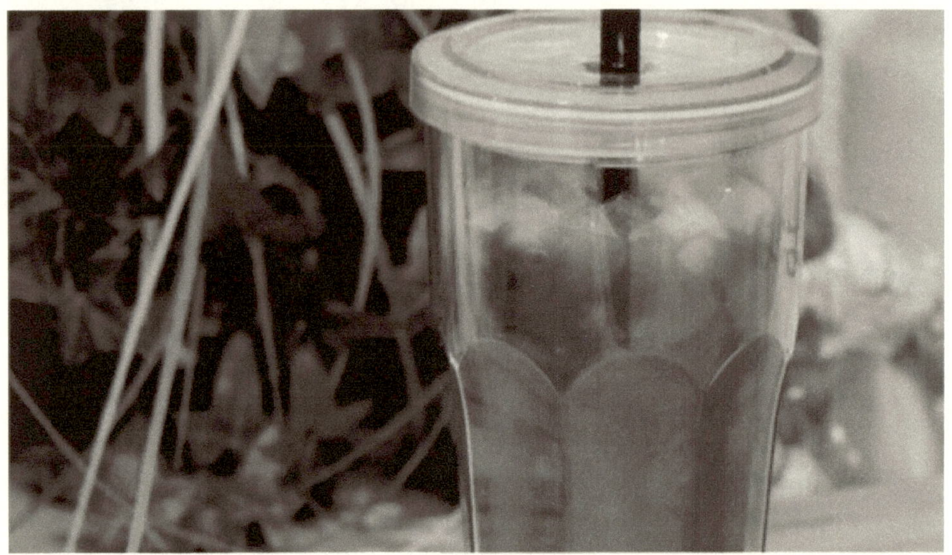

## INGREDIENTS

- 1 1/4 cups cold coffee, divided
- Maxwell House Morning Boost Medium Ground Coffee 30.6 Oz
- 1 envelope low-calorie hot cocoa mix
- 1/2 cup unsweetened almond milk
- 2 tablespoons sugar-free chocolate syrup, or more to taste

# DIRECTIONS

Prep
5 m

Cook
1 m

Ready In
6 m

Servings
1

- Heat 1/4 cup coffee in microwave in a mug until warmed, about 30 seconds. Stir cocoa mix into the coffee until dissolved.
- Fill a large glass with ice cubes. Pour 1 cup cold coffee and almond milk over the ice cubes; stir the cocoa mixture and chocolate syrup into the coffee and almond milk.

# NUTRITION FACTS

Per Serving: 105 calories; 1.8 g fat; 16.7 g carbohydrates; 5.2 g protein; 3 mg cholesterol; 255 mg sodium.

# SPRINGTIME CITRUS COOLER

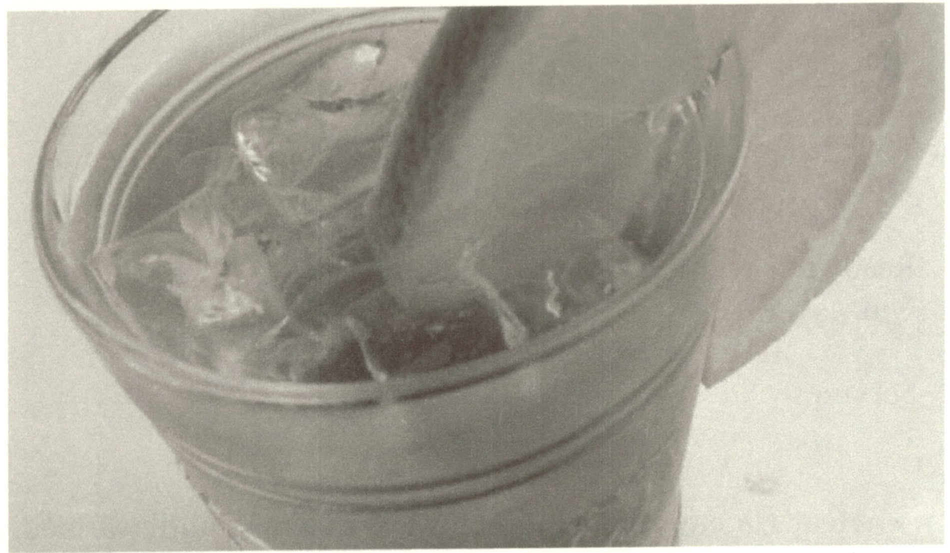

"A springtime and summer favorite in our house, this citrus flavored drink refreshes nicely and serves as a great alternative to tea or water at a brunch."

## INGREDIENTS

- 1 Earl Grey tea bag
- 1 medium orange, thinly sliced
- 3 tablespoons white sugar
- 1 teaspoon rose water (optional)

## DIRECTIONS

Prep
5 m

Cook
5 m

Ready In
10 m

Servings
8

- Prepare a strong cup of tea with the Earl Grey, letting the bag steep for 5 minutes. Place the orange slices, sugar, rose water, and tea into a 1/2 gallon pitcher. Fill with cold water, and stir to dissolve the sugar.

## NUTRITION FACTS

Per Serving: 28 calories; 0 g fat; 7.2 g carbohydrates; 0.2 g protein; 0 mg cholesterol; 0 mg sodium.

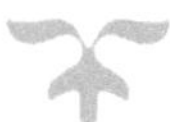

# SOUTH CAROLINA SWEET TEA

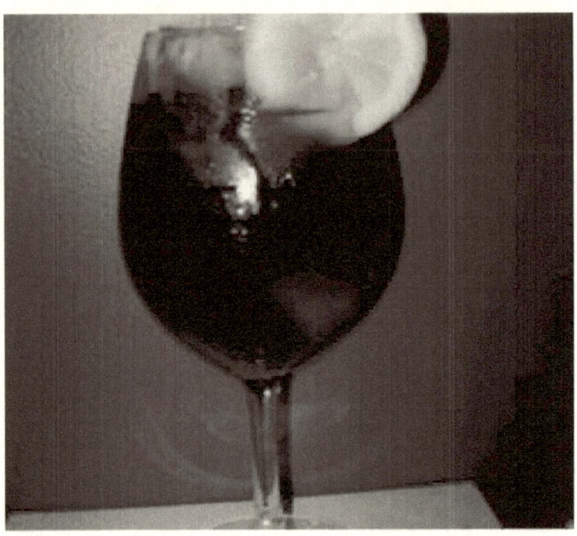

"Remember, this is the South, where simplicity is the secret to most recipes. Follow this to the 'T' and you will have sweet tea, Sand Lapper (South Carolina) style."

## INGREDIENTS

- 3 family size tea bags
- 2 cups white sugar

# DIRECTIONS

Prep
1 m

Cook
10 m

Ready In
11 m

Servings
16

- Using an electric coffee maker, Place the 3 tea bags in the strainer basket (not in the pot). Brew the tea as you would coffee. Pour the sugar in a gallon pitcher. Pour in the hot tea. Continue to run coffee maker with the tea bags until you have enough tea to fill the pitcher. Allow to cool completely at room temperature, then refrigerate.

# NUTRITION FACTS

Per Serving: 97 calories; 0 g fat; 25 g carbohydrates; 0 g protein; 0 mg cholesterol; 0 mg sodium.

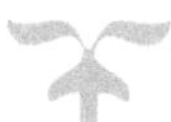

# RUSSIAN TEA II

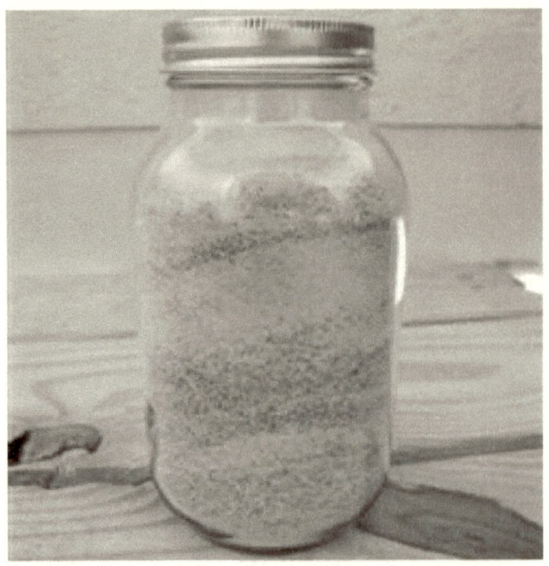

"A great drink for a cold night. You can store this tea mix in a jar and give it as a gift! "

## INGREDIENTS

- 2 cups instant tea with lemon-flavoring dry mix
- 2 cups orange-flavored drink mix
- 1 cup white sugar
- 1 teaspoon ground cinnamon
- 1/2 teaspoon ground cloves

# DIRECTIONS

Prep
5 m

Ready In
5 m

Servings
40

- In a bowl, mix together tea, orange-flavored drink mix, sugar, cinnamon and cloves. To serve place 2 tablespoons mix in a cup and fill with 8 ounces hot water.

# NUTRITION FACTS

Per Serving: 91 calories; 0 g fat; 23.7 g carbohydrates; 0.1 g protein; 0 mg cholesterol; 1 mg sodium.

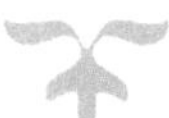

# KUWAITI TRADITIONAL TEA

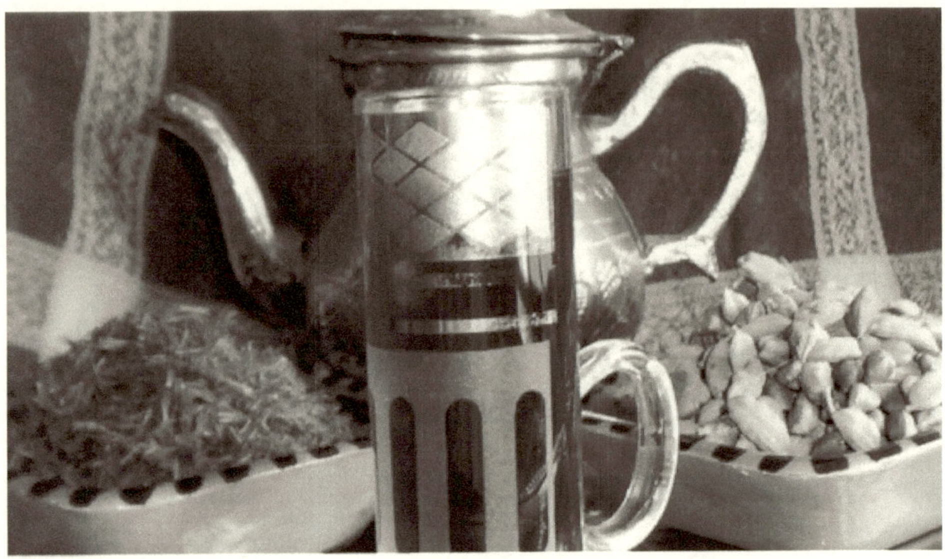

"This is the typical tea you will find in regular housed in Kuwait. Its deliciously aromatic and the spices give it a rich taste."

## INGREDIENTS

- 1 1/2 cups water
- 2 whole cardamom pods, broken
- 1 pinch saffron powder
- 2 tea bags
- 1 teaspoon white sugar (optional)

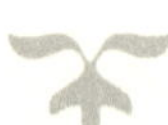

## DIRECTIONS

Prep
2 m

Cook
8 m

Ready In
10 m

Servings
1

- Combine the water, saffron, and cardamom in a saucepan over medium heat. Cover, and bring to a boil. Add tea bags, and let the tea steep for a minute, or longer if you like stronger tea. Strain into a cup, and sweeten with sugar if desired.

## NUTRITION FACTS

Per Serving: 26 calories; 0.1 g fat; 6.2 g carbohydrates; 0.3 g protein; 0 mg cholesterol; 2 mg sodium.

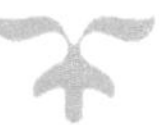